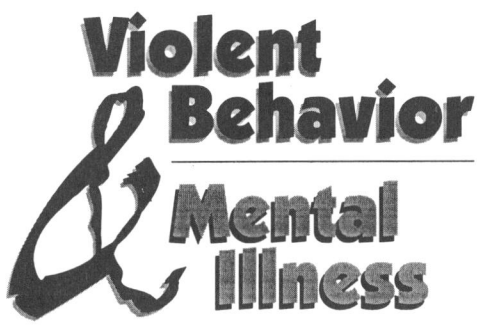

Table of Contents

Introduction
Carl C. Bell, M.D. 2

Putting Violence in Context
Jean Campbell, Ph.D., Susan Stefan, J.D., and Ann Loder 3

Violent Behavior by Individuals With Serious Mental Illness
E. Fuller Torrey, M.D. 4

Assessing the Evidence of a Link Between Mental Illness and Violence
Edward P. Mulvey, Ph.D. 14

Violence and Psychiatric Disorder in the Community: Evidence From the Epidemiologic
Catchment Area Surveys
Jeffrey W. Swanson, Ph.D., Charles E. Holzer III, Ph.D., Vijay K. Ganju, Ph.D.,
and Robert Tsutomu Jono, M.S.P.H. 20

Clinical Symptoms, Neurological Impairment, and Prediction of Violence in Psychiatric Inpatients
Menahem I. Krakowski, M.D., Ph.D., and Pal Czobor, Ph.D. 30

Involuntary Community Treatment of People Who Are Violent and Mentally Ill: A Legal Analysis
Christopher Slobogin, J.D., LL.M. 35

Using Intensive Case Management to Reduce Violence by Mentally Ill Persons
in the Community
Joel A. Dvoskin, Ph.D., and Henry J. Steadman, Ph.D. 40

Pharmacological and Behavioral Treatments for Aggressive Psychiatric Inpatients
Patrick W. Corrigan, Psy.D., Stuart C. Yudofsky, M.D., and Jonathan M. Silver, M.D. 46

The Relationship Between Acute Psychiatric Symptoms, Diagnosis, and Short-Term
Risk of Violence
Dale E. McNiel, Ph.D., and Renée L. Binder, M.D. 55

A Prospective Study of Violence by Psychiatric Patients After Hospital Discharge
Kenneth Tardiff, M.D., M.P.H., Peter M. Marzuk, M.D., Andrew C. Leon, Ph.D., and Laura Portera, B.A. 60

Early-Onset Substance Abuse and Community Violence by Outpatients With Chronic Mental Illness
Carl Fulwiler, M.D., Ph.D., Hillel Grossman, M.D., Catherine Forbes, B.A., and Robin Ruthazer, M.P.H. 64

Command Hallucinations and the Prediction of Dangerousness
John Junginger, Ph.D. 69

Introduction
Carl C. Bell, M.D.

The violence perpetrated by mentally ill patients has not changed much since 1988, when the Hospital and Community Psychiatry Service (now the Psychiatric Services Resource Center) reprinted an outstanding collection of articles from *Hospital and Community Psychiatry* entitled *Management of Violent Behavior*. The majority of articles in that monograph addressed concerns about the immediate response to violence by patients, and they remain relevant today.

However, since 1988 the interactions between mental health professionals, patients (primary consumers), and patient's families (secondary consumers) have changed, and mental health systems are also changing the way they respond to violent behavior by patients. Accordingly, this compendium highlights topics in the current struggle over how to appropriately address the issue of patient violence.

Fortunately, primary and secondary consumers have made great strides in exercising their influence over the mental health system. But while both groups advocate for improvements in system practices, their ideas about what constitute improvements vary, especially when it comes to the system's response to violent patients. Primary consumers are understandably concerned with preserving their rights and ensuring that they are treated with fairness and dignity. However, secondary consumers maintain that they are frequently the victims of violence by patients and advocate for tighter control over them. It is therefore appropriate that the articles in this compendium view advocacy from both perspectives. Other topics germane to the dialogue are also included, such as involuntary community treatment, case management, and psychopharmacology.

Advocates on all sides sometimes overstate their case. Amid all the conflict and controversy over how to deal with violence by mentally ill persons, there is a great need for science that highlights what is known about the problem. Thus this compendium includes articles examining the prevalence of violence and evidence of the link between violent behavior and mental illness. And because researchers fortunately are no longer taking a reductionistic perspective about violence by mentally ill persons, some articles focus on mental states and circumstances in which violence is more likely to occur. Others attempt to identify the small segment of the mentally ill population who are more likely to exhibit chronic violent tendencies.

These articles from *Psychiatric Services* and its predecessor, *Hospital and Community Psychiatry*, are intended to provide some emotional food for thought and some rational scientific findings to guide all of us as we search for the best solution to the problem of patient violence. Ideally, of course, the best solution is to prevent it before it happens. But failing that, taking a systems viewpoint—one that incorporates both science and emotion— seems the most logical approach to developing an appropriate response.

Dr. Bell is president and chief executive officer of the Community Mental Health Council, Inc., in Chicago, clinical professor of psychiatry and public health at the University of Illinois, and a member of Psychiatric Services' *editorial board. In 1997 he was presented with a Special Presidential Commendation by American Psychiatric Association President Harold I. Eist, M.D., for his efforts to reduce violence in America.*

Opinion

Putting Violence in Context

Jean Campbell, Ph.D.
Susan Stefan, J.D.
Ann Loder

We are surrounded by violence: a child is killed by a classmate; a disgruntled employee shoots his boss; a woman is raped and beaten; the inner cities prepare for summer riots. Yet in the midst of local, national, and world violence, communities often focus attention on the dangers that people with mental illness pose to society. A violent act by someone with a history of mental disorders serves as a lightning rod for personal and public fears. Madness has become the generic scapegoat for the evils of modern society.

Fear of the "violent mental patient" permeates all levels of social interaction and provides implicit justification for discrimination. A presumption of violence inevitably isolates an individual from peers and from a community of natural supports. A police officer may more readily shoot a person who has a mental illness; a mother may refuse to allow a mental health consumer to babysit for her child. When someone has a psychiatric diagnosis, anger and joy are routinely scrutinized for signs of pathology.

In fact, people with mental illness are probably more often the victims than the perpetrators of violent crimes. A community residential facility in California was fire-bombed a few years ago by an angry neighbor. A group of youths threw a homeless mentally ill man from a bridge. But who keeps count of these assaults and murders? It becomes the task of mental health consumers and survivors to learn how to live with other people's fear of them. And because of the perceived links between mental illness and violence, individuals can be controlled and coerced in ways unthinkable to the rest of us, including preventive commitment and forced medication.

All these factors underscore the recent findings that violence by persons with a psychiatric diagnosis is grounded in contextual relationships rather than in isolated psychosis. Their lives are set apart by angry or indifferent communities that reject, shun, and sometimes attack them. Sometimes a person's psychotic symptoms can make other people annoyed or afraid, and they may attempt to coerce or control that person in ways that spiral into violence. The contextual nature of violence raises questions of shared culpability, and it challenges taken-for-granted prerogatives of family, clinicians, and agents of community safety to name and manage "the violent mentally ill."

Perhaps the stereotype of the violent, unpredictable mental patient fulfills the social need to situate violence outside "normal" human agency. Only by recognizing that people with mental illness are an integral part of communities scarred by all kinds of violence can we make progress toward a fundamental reassessment of normalcy and human responsibility for evil. ♦

When this commentary was published, Dr. Campbell was with the Maine Department of Mental Health and Mental Retardation in Augusta, Ms. Stefan was with the University of Miami School of Law in Miami, Florida, and Ms. Loder was with the Consumer-Survivor Mental Health Research and Policy Work Group in Fort Lauderdale, Florida. From the July 1994 issue of Hospital and Community Psychiatry *(volume 45, page 633).*

Violent Behavior by Individuals With Serious Mental Illness

E. Fuller Torrey, M.D.

The idea that some individuals with serious mental illness may become violent was prevalent throughout the 19th century. In 1857, for example, Dr. John Gray (1) published an analysis of 49 cases of attempted or completed homicide committed by patients whom he had treated for serious mental illness. Dr. Emil Kraepelin (2) observed in his 1919 treatise on schizophrenia that "in certain circumstances the impulsive actions of the patients may become extraordinarily dangerous." In movies, the stereotype of the mentally ill individual as a "homicidal maniac" can be found as early as *The Maniac Cook* in 1909 (3).

Studies have shown that this stereotype has continued to be widespread. In a 1980 survey of college students' beliefs about individuals with schizophrenia, Wahl (4) found that 52 percent believed that "aggression, hostility, [and] violence" were common or very common attributes, whereas only 9 percent said these attributes were uncommon or very uncommon. A 1987 study of residents of Ohio revealed that "perceived dangerousness" was the single most important factor contributing to the stigma of mental illness (5).

The media have both reflected and propagated this stereotype. In a study of Canadian newspapers between 1977 and 1984, Day (6) found that the traits of dangerousness and unpredictability were commonly attributed to individuals with serious mental illness. Other recent studies have found that newspaper stories tend to specifically link mental illness to crime and that such stories are more likely to be placed on the front page (7). One study of prime-time television indicated that dangerousness and unpredictability were commonly attributed to TV characters who were mentally ill (8). Another study found that 72 percent of mentally ill characters on TV dramas were portrayed as violent (9).

Movies linking mental illness to violence have continued to be popular over the years; examples of this genre include *Psycho, Repulsion, Friday the 13th, Halloween,* and *Nightmare on Elm Street* and, more recently, *Silence of the Lambs* and *Single White Female.*

Stigmatization and negative stereotypes create major problems for individuals with serious mental illness and their families, making access to housing, jobs, social programs, and

Objective: *The perceived association between violent behavior and serious mental illness was explored to determine the validity of claims by mental health advocates that individuals with serious mental illness are no more dangerous than members of the general population.* **Methods:** *The author reviewed recent studies and media accounts of violent behavior by individuals with serious mental illness, with emphasis given to the most recent studies.* **Results and conclusions:** *Although the vast majority of individuals with serious mental illness are not more dangerous than members of the general population, recent findings suggest the existence of a subgroup that is more dangerous. A history of violent behavior, noncompliance with medications, and substance abuse are important predictors of violent behavior in this subgroup. The findings imply that the criteria for involuntary hospitalization, involuntary medication, outpatient commitment, the monitoring of medication compliance, and other mandated follow-up procedures may need to be revised. The existence of a subgroup of seriously mentally ill patients who exhibit violent behavior undermines efforts by mental health advocates to reduce the stigma of mental illness by denying an association with violence. Until the problem of violence by this subgroup is addressed, it will be difficult to substantially decrease the stigma associated with serious mental illness.*

When this paper was published **Dr. Torrey** *was a guest researcher at the National Institute of Mental Health Neuroscience Center at St. Elizabeths Hospital in Washington, D.C. From the July 1994 issue of* Hospital and Community Psychiatry *(vlume. 45, pages 653–662).*

even psychiatric care more difficult. In fact, some individuals with a serious mental illness say that the stigma is worse than the disease itself. For this reason, the National Alliance for the Mentally Ill (NAMI) and the National Stigma Clearinghouse operated by the Alliance for the Mentally Ill of New York State have made concerted efforts in recent years to combat the stigma and negative stereotypes connected with serious mental illness. The link between serious mental illness and violent behavior has also been questioned by some writers who assert that "a mentally ill person is not significantly more likely than anyone else to be violent" (10). Because destigmatizing these illnesses depends on public understanding of the connection between serious mental illness and violent behavior, it is important to examine the data on this association.

This paper reviews objective studies and media stories on violence and mental illness, with emphasis given to the most recent studies. The literature review is followed by a discussion of factors that contribute to violent behavior by individuals with serious mental illness and recommendations for policy changes designed to increase public safety and decrease the stigma of serious mental illness.

Studies of violent behavior

The incidence of violent behavior among individuals with serious mental illness has been examined through studies of five different groups: individuals who have been arrested, psychiatric inpatients, psychiatric outpatients, families with a member who has a serious mental illness, and individuals identified as having a serious mental illness by surveys of the general population. Each of these groups contributes a different perspective to the problem.

Individuals who have been arrested. The arrest rate of individuals who have a serious mental illness has been the most commonly used measure of their dangerousness. Studies done in 1922, 1930, 1938, and 1945 all found "that mentally ill persons had a lower arrest rate than the general population" (11) and led to the oft-quoted claim that mentally ill individuals are

Since the advent of deinstitutionalization in the 1960s, studies of individuals with a serious mental illness have found their arrest rate is substantially higher than that of the general population.

no more dangerous than other people. A reason for this belief may be that those studies took place during a time when individuals with serious mental illness were routinely confined to psychiatric hospitals for much of their adult lives.

Since the advent of deinstitutionalization in the 1960s, studies of individuals with a serious mental illness have found their arrest rate is substantially higher than that of the general population. A 1992 survey of 1,391 American jails reported that 7.2 percent of the inmates had manifest symptoms of schizophrenia or bipolar disorder (12). Methodologically, the best studies of mentally ill individuals in jails were done by Teplin (13) in Chicago (6.4 percent of jail admissions had schizophrenia, mania, or major depression) and Guy and colleagues (14) in Philadelphia (14.4 percent of jail admissions had schizophrenia or mania). Other studies have reported percentages that fall between these estimates (12).

Studies of state prisons have also reported that inmates with schizophrenia and bipolar disorder constitute a substantial minority of the population. In a review of these studies, Jemelka and others (15) concluded that 10 to 15 percent of prison populations have a major *DSM-III-R* thought disorder or mood disorder and need the services usually associated with severe or chronic mental illnesses.

Arrest rates alone, however, are not good indexes of violent behavior because most arrests are for nonviolent offenses. This is especially true for individuals with a serious mental illness, among whom arrests for misdemeanors such as trespassing and disorderly conduct are very common (12). A study in Alaska found that only 28 percent of the arrests of referred schizophrenic patients were for violent crimes (16). The Alaskan study also estimated that 1 percent of all persons with schizophrenia in Alaska were arrested for violent crimes each year (16).

Lamb and Grant (17) did studies in the Los Angeles County jail of the types of crimes committed by individuals with a serious mental illness. Among 96 male inmates referred for psychiatric evaluation, 43 had been charged with misdemeanors and 53 with felonies. Among those charged with felonies, 27 inmates (28 percent of the total group) had been charged with violent crimes (nine with armed robbery, eight with assault with a deadly weapon, four with murder, two with assault on a peace officer, two with felony assault, and two with rape). A similar study of 97 female inmates referred for psychiatric evaluation found that 60 had been charged with misdemeanors and 37 with felonies, including 17 (18 percent of the total group) with violent crimes (18).

Another approach to this problem is to study the psychiatric status of individuals charged with particular types of violent crime. Martell and Dietz (19) identified 36 individuals who had pushed or tried to push other people in front of subway trains in New York City. Twenty-five of the 36 were referred for psychiatric evaluation, and data were available on 20 of them. Fourteen had a diagnosis of schizophrenia (eight had the paranoid subtype); one, schizoaffective disorder; one, bipolar disorder; three, psychosis not otherwise specified; and one, antisocial personality disorder. Except for one episode that took place during an attempted robbery, the authors found that all of the motives reported by these offenders reflected psychotic symptoms. Thus individuals with serious mental illnesses appear to be responsible for the majority of cases of this particular type of violent crime.

Psychiatric inpatients. Numerous studies have been made of violent acts committed by mentally ill persons before admission, during the course of hospitalization, and following discharge from psychiatric hospitals. Studies of acts committed before admission and during hospitalization are of limited usefulness because violent acts are a major selection criterion for psychiatric hospital admission and because psychiatric ward personnel and policies may influence the number of violent acts committed by patients. Studies of discharged patients are more useful and in fact should err on the side of minimizing the problem of violent behavior because patients are usually not discharged until they no longer are considered potentially violent.

Several studies of individuals discharged from psychiatric hospitals have been done since deinstitutionalization. Studies before 1979 were reviewed by Rabkin (20), who concluded that "over the past 20 years, mental patients discharged from public facilities as a group have total arrest rates for all crimes that equal or exceed public rates with which they have been compared. Arrest and conviction rates for the subcategory of violent crimes were found to exceed general population rates in every study in which they were measured."

A more recent study by Klassen and O'Connor (21) reported that 25 to 30 percent of male psychiatric patients with a history of violent behavior became violent again within one year after discharge. Another recent study found that 27 percent of released male and female patients reported at least one violent act within a mean of four months after discharge (22).

Shore and others (23), in a study of hospitalized "White House cases" (individuals, usually with schizophrenia, who present themselves at the White House to see the President for delusional reasons), reported that following discharge, subjects with a history of prior arrests had a threefold higher rate of subsequent arrests for murder, assault, or robbery than did subjects without prior arrests or a control population. Similar findings also emerged from a Swedish study of 644 individuals with schizophrenia who were followed for 15 years after their initial psychiatric hospitalization, a period during which they committed four times more violent offenses than did a normal control population (24).

Studies such as these led the late Dr. Saleem Shah (25) of the National Institute of Mental Health to write in 1990 that "almost every large study since the sixties has found that persons with histories of mental hospitalization (typically in public sector facilities) tend to have subsequent arrest rates higher than those for the general population."

Psychiatric outpatients. In addition to the postdischarge studies of psychiatric inpatients cited above, three studies of violent behavior among psychiatric outpatients have been done. In the first, conducted in New Hampshire by Bartels and others (26), 133 outpatients with a diagnosis of schizophrenia were rated on a 5-point scale, with 1 indicating no hostility; 2, irritability and argumentativeness; 3, verbally threatening behavior or mild object-directed aggression; 4, destruction of property or interpersonal assault without harm; and 5, assaultiveness with potential or actual harm.

Of the 133 outpatients, three were rated as being assaultive with potential or actual harm, 14 as being destructive of property or assaultive without harm, 24 as verbally threatening or having mild object-related aggression, 28 as irritable and argumentative, and 64 as showing no hostility. Higher levels of hostility were significantly correlated with being male and with having a diagnosis of schizoaffective disorder. There was also a strong correlation between hostility and medication compliance: 71 percent of the outpatients rated as assaultive or destructive of property had problems with medication compliance, compared with only 17 percent of those rated at level 1 (p<.001). Furthermore, higher levels of hostility strongly predicted rehospitalization of the individual within one year (p=.002).

Another American study of violent behavior in psychiatric outpatients was reported by Link and colleagues (27) in New York. They compared 186 outpatients and 46 inpatients with 521 community residents who had not received any psychiatric care. Methodologically, it is probably the best study done to date on violent behavior in psychiatric patients; the groups were matched on a wide variety of demographic characteristics, and violent behavior was measured in multiple ways (arrests, hitting others, fighting, weapon use, and "hurting someone badly"). The group of psychiatric patients was further divided into first-contact patients, who had begun treatment within the past year; repeat-treatment patients, who had begun treatment more than a year previously and were currently being treated; and former patients, who had been treated in the past but not within the previous year.

The psychiatric patients were found to have engaged in significantly more violent behavior than the community residents. Results for the two most important indicators of violence, weapon use in the past five years and hurting someone badly, are summarized in Table 1. They show that in comparison with the other community residents, the psychiatric patients were two to three times more likely to have exhibited violent behavior.

The Link study found that no demographic and socioeconomic variables accounted for the differences in

Table 1

Percentage of participants exhibiting two types of violent behavior in a study by Link and colleagues (72)

Group	Weapon use (past five years)	Hurting someone badly (lifetime)
Community residents	2.7	5.4
Psychiatric patients		
First contact	2.1	18.8**
Repeat treatment	11.7	12.9**
Former patients	11.1*	16.7*

*p<.05
**p<.01

Table 2

Percentage of respondents in the Epidemiologic Catchment Area study who reported four types of violent behavior in the past year

Diagnosis	Hit parner	Hit child	Fought with others	Used weapon
No psychiatric disorder (N=7,379)	0.6	0.1	0.8	0.4
Serious mental illness (N=426)				
Schizophrenia or schizophreniform disorder (N=114)	5.3	0.8	6.9	8.6
Bipolar disorder (N=30)	5.3	2.1	0	0
Major depression (N=282)	5.2	1.2	4.8	5.0

violent behavior between the two groups. The only variable that did account for the differences was the current level of psychotic symptoms; that is, the sicker the patients, the more likely they were to have exhibited violent behavior.

Similar findings were reported in a recent English study of 538 individuals with schizophrenia living in the Camberwell district of London (28). Individuals with psychiatric diagnoses other than schizophrenia, matched for age and sex with the study group, were used as control subjects. In comparison with the control subjects, male schizophrenic patients were found to have a 3.9 times greater risk and female schizophrenic patients a 5.3 times greater risk for conviction on charges of assault and serious violence.

The potential for violence by outpatients with serious mental illness is a threat that is also familiar to mental health professionals who work with such patients. In recent years there have been several assaults on professionals by outpatients who had serious mental illness, including at least three that were fatal (29–31).

Families with a seriously ill member. In 1990 the National Alliance for the Mentally Ill made an extensive study of 1,401 families in which a family member had a serious mental illness (32). In almost all cases, the ill family member had a diagnosis of schizophrenia, bipolar disorder, or major depression. The researchers reported that within the preceding year, 10.6 percent of the individuals with a serious mental illness had physically harmed another person, and another 12.2 percent had threatened to harm another person.

The study found a marked sex difference among those threatening harm (24.9 percent of males and 12.5 percent of females) but surprisingly little sex difference among those actually harming someone (11.9 percent of males and 9.5 percent of females). An earlier survey of NAMI families had found that more than one-third of the families reported that their ill relative was assaultive and destructive in the home either sometimes or frequently (33).

The results of the NAMI surveys are consistent with other reports of violence against family members by individuals with serious mental illness. Straznickas and colleagues (34) reported that among patients admitted to psychiatric hospitals who had physically attacked someone within the preceding two weeks, family members had been the object of the assault 56 percent of the time. A similar study by Tardiff (35) reported that family members had been the object of the assault 65 percent of the time. Previous surveys of problems encountered by families with a seriously mentally ill relative living at home have also reported threatening or assaultive behavior as a common problem (36).

The results of the NAMI surveys are also consistent with anecdotal reports of violence against family members by individuals with a serious mental illness (37–39). A frequent theme in these accounts is the association between the violence and the mentally ill individual's refusal to take medication; for example, in an article entitled "My Brother Might Kill Me," the author wrote that her brother's last several attacks all took place following his refusal to take his medication (40). The psychological as well as physical trauma that these family members sustain was summarized by one mother who had been the object of an attack: "The thought of being attacked and physically harmed by another is frightening in itself, but when the attacker is your own flesh and blood, it is additional, unspeakable trauma upon trauma as your whole being sways between love and fear" (41).

Surveys of the general population. Two studies have been done of violent behavior among individuals with serious mental illnesses who were identified by surveys of the general population. As such, the individuals in these studies were not selected in any way by treatment criteria or by having been arrested.

The first study was the five-site Epidemiologic Catchment Area (ECA) surveys, carried out between 1980 and 1983 by the National Institute of Mental Health (42). The survey assessed violence by using four criteria: hitting or throwing things at one's wife, husband, or partner; hitting one's child hard enough to cause bruises or injury; physical fighting with others; and using a weapon such as a stick, knife, or gun in a fight. A major shortcoming of the study was the lack of ratings for the severity of the violent behavior; hitting someone with a stick and killing someone with a gun were rated equally.

The results, summarized in Table 2, show that individuals with a serious mental illness living in the community reported having been violent within the previous year much more frequently than individuals who had no mental disorder. The frequency with which individuals with schizophrenia reported having used a weapon in a fight (21.5 times more often than individuals with no psychiatric disorder) is especially noteworthy. In addition, the study found that almost one-third of the individuals with schizophrenia or schizophreniform disorder also met diagnostic criteria for drug or alcohol abuse or dependence and that these individuals had a much higher rate of reported violence than did those without this co-factor. Higher rates of reported violence were found among individuals who had drug or alcohol abuse or dependence and no serious mental illness than among individuals with serious mental illness alone.

The other random community survey, done in Sweden (43), included all individuals born in Stockholm in 1953 and still living there 30 years later. The study focused on violent crimes committed by individuals with a serious mental disorder. Violent crimes were defined as including "all offenses involving the use of threat of physical violence (for example, assault, rape, robbery, unlawful threat, and molestation)." Major mental disorder was defined as including schizophrenia, paranoid states, major affective disorders, and other psychoses. In comparison with men and women with no psychiatric diagnoses, men with major mental disorders were found to be 4.2 times more likely and women with major mental disorders 27.5 times more likely to have been convicted of a violent crime.

Media accounts of violent behavior

In addition to the objective studies reviewed above, it is useful to examine media accounts of violent behavior by individuals with serious mental illness. Although the media do not use scientific methodology in the selection of their subjects, they reflect events in the community and also shape public opinion about these events. As Steadman (44) has noted, "What the public knows about how the mentally ill behave is for the most part garnered from newspaper reports, television and radio news, and television dramatizations."

Isolated examples of media coverage of mentally ill individuals who commit violent acts can be found throughout this century. Among the most highly publicized episodes in the years following World War II were the 13 murders committed by Howard Unruh in Camden, New Jersey, in 1949 (45); the 13 murders committed by Herbert Mullin in the San Francisco Bay area in 1972 (46); and the multiple spree of rapes, robberies, and murders of Joseph Kallinger ("The Shoemaker") in the Philadelphia area in 1974 (47). All three men were diagnosed as having schizophrenia.

In recent years, however, reports of violence by individuals with serious mental illness have become commonplace. Some highly publicized examples of such reports for each year since 1980 follow.

1980: In New York, Dennis Sweeney, diagnosed as having paranoid schizophrenia, killed Congressman Allard Lowenstein, who Sweeney believed was causing his auditory hallucinations (48).

1981: In Washington, D.C., John Hinckley, diagnosed as having schizophrenia, shot President Reagan and three others (49).

1982: In Tokyo, a pilot for Japan Air Lines, responding to auditory hallucinations, crashed an airliner into Tokyo Bay (50).

1983: In California, Michael Miller, a young man with schizophrenia who was the son of President Reagan's tax attorney, killed his mother (51).

1984: In California, Henry Lucas, a drifter who had been diagnosed as having schizophrenia, was charged with the murder of 36 women (52).

1985: In Philadelphia, Sylvia Seegrist, diagnosed as having schizophrenia, killed three people and wounded seven others in a shooting spree in a shopping mall (53).

1986: In New York, Juan Gonzalez, diagnosed as having schizophrenia, killed two and wounded nine others on the Staten Island ferry in an attack with a sword (54).

1987: In Michigan, Bartley Dobben, diagnosed as psychotic, killed his two young sons by putting them into a foundry ladle (55).

1988: In Chicago, Laurie Dann, diagnosed as having schizophrenia, killed one child and wounded five others in an attack in a school classroom (56).

1989: In Louisville, Joseph Wesbecker, diagnosed as having bipolar disorder, killed seven coworkers and wounded 13 others (57).

1990: In Atlanta, James Brady, who was diagnosed as having schizophrenia and who believed he was being controlled by a machine in his body, killed one person and wounded four others in a shooting spree in a shopping center (58).

1991: In California, Philip Jablonski, who had a diagnosis of schizophrenia and past convictions for rape and murder, killed four more women within seven months after his release from prison (59).

1992: In New York, Larry Hogue, diagnosed as having chronic psychosis and a drug abuse disorder, was involuntarily hospitalized after attempting to injure residents of a Manhattan neighborhood (60).

1993: In Alabama, Eileen Janezic, diagnosed as having bipolar disorder, was charged with the murder of a minister and the shooting of another man. At the time of her arrest she was carrying the "Satanic Bible"(61).

These examples include only incidents in which individuals with a serious mental illness attacked other people. They do not include cases not involving assault, such as the 1986 case in which Randall Husar used a hammer to smash the glass case that holds the Constitution and the Bill of Rights in Washington, D.C. (62), or the 1990 case in which Stephen Blumberg was arrested in Iowa for stealing approximately 11,000 rare books from libraries (63), or the 1992 case in which Patrick Lee Frank was indicted for setting 20 church fires in Tennessee and Florida (64). All three men had been diagnosed as having schizophrenia. Nor do they include other highly publicized but less serious assaults, such as the man "muttering about earthquakes and revelations" who, without warning, punched Senator John Glenn during a 1989 public tree-planting ceremony (65).

In reviewing these and other media accounts of violent acts by individuals with serious mental illness, three aspects stand out. First, most of the perpetrators of the violent acts had previously been under psychiatric care. Indeed, in many cases the seriously mentally ill individual had been evaluated and released by a psychiatrist within days or even hours of the act.

Second, women with serious mental illness appear to commit almost as many violent acts as do men with serious mental illness. This phenomenon is in sharp contrast to violent acts committed by individuals who are not mentally ill, the vast majority of which are committed by men.

Third, media accounts of violent acts by mentally ill individuals appear to have increased in frequency since approximately 1980 and seem to be continuing to increase. Such an increase would be consonant with many of the studies discussed previously, including one study that specifically reported an increasing incidence of violent behavior by mentally ill individuals (66).

It is, of course, not possible to use media sources as a means of quantifying violent acts by individuals with serious mental illness because it is not known how many of the total number of such acts are discovered and reported by the media. However, to assess the number of acts that do come to media attention, the author collected all such examples reported during one year (1992) in a single newspaper, the *Washington Post*, which covers the Washington, D.C., metropolitan area of approximately three million people. The examples included the following.

♦ Jayant Vatz, diagnosed as having bipolar disorder and responding to "a thousand voices," pleaded guilty to the murder of his father and stepmother (67).

♦ Sandra Moneymaker, said to have "severe depression with psychotic features," was found innocent by reason of insanity in the killing of her two sons (68).

♦ Kathlynn Najeera, suffering from "acute paranoid schizophrenia," was found insane and was committed to a mental hospital after she intentionally drove her car into and killed a ten-year-old boy on a bicycle (69).

♦ Brian Bechtold, diagnosed as having paranoid schizophrenia, was said to be legally insane at the time he killed his mother and father (70).

♦ Alan Newman, arrested and suspected of being responsible for five homicides, had previously been found to be "acutely psychotic" and "characteristically quite disturbed" by a psychiatrist (71).

♦ Hadden Clark, who killed a young woman in her home, had been twice diagnosed as having schizophrenia (72).

These reported incidents reflect coverage of a population of approximately three million people. If they could be extrapolated to the population of the country, there would have been a total of approximately 500 similar incidents reported by newspapers in the United States in 1992.

Discussion

It is a well-documented fact that America is a violent society. Of the 19 million crime victimizations reported in 1990, nearly one-third involved violence (73). Within this broad landscape of violence, the contribution of individuals with a serious mental illness to the total picture is not large. This situation stands in contrast to less violent societies, such as Iceland, in which only 47 homicides were committed over 80 years, but individuals with serious mental illness were responsible for 13 (28 percent) of them (74). Alcohol and drug abusers in the United States are as a group much more violent than individuals with serious mental illness.

The studies reviewed above verify the fact that the vast majority of individuals with serious mental illness are not violent and are not more dangerous than individuals in the general population. A subgroup of such individuals, however, is more dangerous, and the data suggest that this problem is increasing. The findings that 27 percent of released male and female psychiatric patients report at least one violent act within a mean of four months after discharge (22), that 8.6 percent of individuals with schizophrenia living in the community had used a weapon in a fight within the preceding year (42), and that 10.6 percent of individuals with serious mental illness had physically harmed another within the preceding year (32) should be of concern to all mental health professionals.

As summarized by Dr. John Monahan (22) after his review of such studies, "The data that have recently become available, fairly read, suggest the one conclusion I did not want to reach . . . there appears to be a relationship between mental disorder and violent behavior." Because there are by conservative estimates approximately 2.5 million individuals with schizophrenia or bipolar disorder in the United States, the total number of violent acts being committed by these individuals is of great concern.

Insofar as there is a relationship between violent behavior and a subgroup within the population of individuals with serious mental illness, the public stereotype that links violence with mental illness is based on reality and not merely on stigma. Therefore, present attempts to combat this stereotype by campaigns of public education will fail until the problem of violent behavior is addressed.

Lagos and associates (75) noted this fact as early as 1977 in an article entitled "Fear of the Mentally Ill: Empirical Support for the Common Man's Response." In 1981 Steadman (44) similarly observed that "recent research data on contemporary populations of ex-mental patients supports these public fears [of dangerousness] to an extent rarely acknowledged by mental health professionals. . . . It is [therefore] futile and inappropriate to badger the news and entertainment media with appeals to help destigmatize the mentally ill." In a similar vein, Monahan (22) recently added, "The data suggest that public education programs by advocates for the mentally disordered along the lines of 'people with mental illness are no more violent than the rest of us' may be doomed to failure. . . . And they should: the claim, it turns out, may well be untrue." Currently, then, the average citizen may ride to work on a bus that has a poster proclaiming mentally ill individuals are not dangerous, while he or she reads that day's newspaper headline saying in effect that some of them are dangerous.

Considering that violent acts are committed by a small minority within the population of seriously mentally ill persons, are there indicators from the studies that suggest which individuals are likely to be violent? One strong predictor, applicable to all individuals, is a history of violent behavior. Another strong predictor, also applicable to everyone, is concurrent alcohol or drug abuse. For those with serious mental illness, concurrent alcohol or drug abuse may be an even stronger predictor of violent behavior because substance abuse exacerbates symptoms in many individuals.

A third factor that appears to be an important predictor is noncompliance with medication. It is known that there are a variety of reasons why those who are mentally ill do not take medication, including lack of insight, medication side effects, and a poor doctor-patient relationship. It is also known that individuals with serious mental illness have a high failure rate in taking medication; in one study, only 50 percent were still taking prescribed antipsychotic medication one year after hospital discharge (76).

Individuals who do not take prescribed medication appear to be much more likely to commit violent acts. For example, in the study of psychiatric outpatients by Bartels and colleagues (26), "71 percent of the violent patients . . . had problems with medication compliance, compared with only 17 percent of those without hostile behaviors," and the correlation was highly significant (p<.001).

Similarly, in a study of inmates in a state forensic hospital, Smith (77) found a highly significant correlation (p<.001) between failure to take medication and history of violent acts in the community. Another measure of failure to take prescribed antipsychotic medication is continuing prominent psychotic symptoms, because taking medication reduces such symptoms in most cases. In the study by Link and others (27) of individuals with serious mental illness who were living in the community, psychotic symptoms were highly correlated with fighting (p<.001) and hitting others (p<.01), and they were "the only variable that accounts for differences in levels of violent illegal behavior between patients and never-treated community residents."

A similar association of psychotic symptoms and violent acts was reported by Taylor (78) in her English study of 121 men with psychosis who had committed crimes. She concluded that "over 80 percent of the offenses of the psychotic [men] were probably attributable to their illness. . . . Within the psychotic group those driven to offend by their delusions were most likely to have been seriously violent, and psychotic symptoms probably accounted directly for most of the very violent behavior."

Studies of psychiatric inpatients have also consistently shown correlations between insufficient medication

It should be remembered that violent behavior by individuals with serious mental illness is merely one aspect of a larger problem—the failure of public psychiatric services and deinstitutionalization.

and increased violent behavior (79–81).

At an anecdotal level, there is also support for believing that the failure to take medication is an important predictor of violent behavior in individuals with serious mental illness. Phrases such as "he had gone a long time without his medication" [when he killed his mother] (82) and "his daughter was not taking her medication at the time of the slaying" [of her mother] (83) recur regularly in newspaper accounts of such violent acts. The data, then, suggest that individuals with serious mental illnesses are *not* more dangerous than the general population *when they are taking their antipsychotic medication.* When they are not taking their medication, the existing data suggest that some of them are more dangerous.

The fact that many individuals with serious mental illness do not take the prescribed medication that they need to control their psychotic symptoms is not unexpected. The brain, the organ that we use for insight and appreciation of our needs, is the same organ whose function is impaired by schizophrenia and bipolar disorder. Recent studies of insight have shown it to be severely impaired in many individuals with serious mental illness.

A study by David and others (84; David A, personal communication, 1992) in London found that 47 percent of inpatients with psychosis scored between 0 and 8 on an 18-point scale of insight. Amador and Strauss (85) in New York reported that nearly 60 percent of the patients with schizophrenia had "moderate to severe unawareness" of having a mental disorder. Amador and associates (86) also reviewed studies relating insight to medication compliance and reported that the bulk of the evidence supports a direct relationship between the two. Calling lack of insight the "core problem" of mentally ill homeless individuals, the *Wall Street Journal* said "that problem, simply put, is that the mentally ill require treatment which they are incapable of seeking for themselves" (87).

In addition to history of violence, concurrent substance abuse, and medication noncompliance, previous studies have suggested other possible predictors of violence in individuals with serious mental illness. Delusions, especially those in which people believe that someone or something has taken control of their mind, have been found to be correlated with violent behavior in studies in England (88). Neurological impairment is also found more commonly in mentally ill individuals who are violent (89), and there has been speculation about whether some violent mentally ill individuals may have a form of epilepsy that has not been diagnosed. Command hallucinations are also frequently cited as predictors of violent behavior.

Is it possible to predict which seriously mentally ill individuals will become violent? Studies done in the 1970s reported that mental health professionals were unable to predict violence in their patients at more than a chance level. A recent reanalysis of those studies by Apperson, Mulvey, Lidz, and Gardner (90, 91) demonstrated flawed methodology in many of the earlier studies (90) and concluded that "clinical judgment has been undervalued in previous research" (91). Using all the predictive factors enumerated above, it may be possible to predict violent behavior in individuals with serious mental illness at a clinically useful level. An important longitudinal study of risk assessment in individuals with serious mental illness, funded by the MacArthur Foundation, is now under way in Pittsburgh, Worcester, Massachusetts, and Kansas City but will not be completed until 1995 (92).

Finally, it should be remembered that violent behavior by individuals with serious mental illness is merely one aspect of a larger problem—the failure of public psychiatric services and deinstitutionalization. Other aspects of this problem include the large number of individuals with a serious mental illness among the homeless (93); the large number of individuals with a serious mental illness in jails and prisons (12,15); and the revolving door of psychiatric hospital readmissions, through which it becomes necessary to readmit 30 percent of patients within 30 days after discharge (94), with some individuals accumulating more than 100 readmissions (95).

Recommendations

The fact that some individuals with serious mental illness, especially those who are not taking prescribed medications, are more prone to acts of violence has important implications for mental health services. Theoretically, many such acts are preventable with good medication compliance and assertive case management. One Canadian study found that under such conditions, discharged patients with serious mental illness had a comparatively low incidence of violent acts (96).

The following are several steps that can be taken to decrease the incidence of violent acts by seriously mentally ill individuals.

♦ Criteria for involuntary psychiatric hospitalization should incorporate the most important predictors of dangerousness, such as medication noncompliance, history of violent behavior, and concurrent drug and alcohol abuse. In many states, the laws specifying dangerousness currently restrict such consideration to acts occurring only within the previous 30 days. This restriction is at variance with what is known about recurrent violent acts in such individuals and with the remitting and relapsing course of these illnesses.

♦ The right to involuntarily medicate a patient should be automatically included with the right to involuntarily hospitalize a patient. The current situation in many states, in which a person with serious mental illness can be involuntarily hospitalized but not involuntarily medicated, makes no sense.

♦ Outpatient commitment, in which an individual with serious mental illness can remain in the community only as long as he or she takes medication and otherwise complies with specified treatment, should be used much more widely. The majority of states have laws allowing for outpatient commitment, but they are remarkably underused. In some states, a person with tuberculosis and schizophrenia may be treated involuntarily for the tuberculosis but not for the schizophrenia (97).

♦ Individuals with serious mental illness who have a history of violent behavior should not be released into the community from hospitals, jails, or prisons unless provisions have been made and monitoring is in place to ensure that they will continue to take prescribed medication. The current situation in most states is both troubling and unknown to the general public. For example, Lamb (98) followed up 85 men with serious mental illness who had been jailed for serious crimes (11 for murder or attempted murder, 14 for armed robbery, 19 for assault with a deadly weapon, three for rape, ten for burglary, and 28 for other crimes). Two-thirds of the men had been convicted of a previous felony. At the end of two years, 36 percent were still incarcerated and 26 percent had been released on probation, but 38 percent had been simply released, with no plan whatsoever for monitoring or follow-up. Oregon's Psychiatric Security Review Board is considered to be a model program for providing continuing oversight for such individuals (99).

♦ Mechanisms should be developed to monitor compliance with oral medication schedules among patients who have a serious mental illness and a history of violent behavior. At present, only injectable medications (fluphenazine, haloperidol) and oral lithium can be monitored, lithum by measuring blood levels. Substances that are detectable in the urine, such as small amounts of isioniazid or riboflavin, have been mixed with medications and successfully used to monitor medication compliance for diseases such as tuberculosis and leprosy (100,101). These substances could also be used for monitoring oral medication needed to control the symptoms of serious mental illnesses.

Implementing these recommendations would require changes in some state laws that would be opposed by many civil libertarians. However, given the overwhelming evidence that some individuals who have a serious mental illness are violent and therefore a danger to other people, it is important to balance the rights of other community residents with the rights of those with a serious mental illness.

Some think the public at large would be more willing than the mental health or legal communities to make the necessary changes. For example, the *New York Times,* a dependable defender of civil liberties, recently published an article entitled "The West Side Has Lost Patience" (102). It described "a child being wheeled in a carriage on Broadway [who] was slapped by a deranged man" and "a deranged man who tried to bite [a man's] leg." The article then concluded, "We have, sadly, grown accustomed to the images of madness on our streets and the menacing life that lives on them and now owns them." ♦

References

1. Gray JP: Homicide in insanity. American Journal of Insanity 14:119–143, 1857
2. Kraepelin E: Dementia Praecox and Paraphrenia. Huntington, NY, Robert Krieger, 1971 (originally published in 1919)
3. Hyler SE, Gabbard GO, Schneider I: Movie madness. Journal of the California Alliance for the Mentally Ill 4:4–7, 1993
4. Wahl OF: Public vs professional conceptions of schizophrenia. Journal of Community Psychology 15:285–291, 1987
5. Link BG, Cullen FT, Frank J, et al: The social rejection of former mental patients: understanding why labels matter. American Journal of Sociology 92:1461–1500, 1987
6. Day DM: Portrayal of mental illness in Canadian newspapers. Canadian Journal of Psychiatry 31:813–816, 1986
7. Wahl O: Mass media images of mental illness: a review of the literature. Journal of Community Psychology 20:343–352, 1992
8. Wahl OF, Roth R: Television images of

mental illness: results of a metropolitan Washington media watch. Journal of Broadcasting 28:599–605, 1982

9. Signorelli N: The stigma of mental illness on television. Journal of Broadcasting and Electronic Media 33:325–331, 1989

10. Trafford A: For the mentally ill, another stigma. Washington Post, Jan 5, 1988, p A17

11. Brown P: The Transfer of Care: Psychiatric Deinstitutionalization and Its Aftermath. London, Routledge & Kegan Paul, 1985

12. Torrey EF, Stieber J, Ezekiel J, et al: Criminalizing the Seriously Mentally Ill: The Abuse of Jails as Mental Hospitals. Washington, DC, National Alliance for the Mentally Ill and Public Citizen's Health Research Group, 1992

13. Teplin LA: The prevalence of severe mental disorder among male urban jail detainees: comparison with Epidemiologic Catchment Area Program. American Journal of Public Health 80:639–669, 1990

14. Guy E, Platt JJ, Zwerling I, et al: Mental health status of prisoners in an urban jail. Criminal Justice and Behavior 12:29–53, 1985

15. Jemelka R, Trupin E, Chiles JA: The mentally ill in prisons. Hospital and Community Psychiatry 40:481–485, 1989

16. Phillips MR, Wolf AS, Coons DJ: Psychiatry and the criminal justice system: testing the myths. American Journal of Psychiatry 145:605–610, 1988

17. Lamb HR, Grant RW: The mentally ill in an urban county jail. Archives of General Psychiatry 39:17–22, 1982

18. Lamb HR, Grant RW: Mentally ill women in a county jail. Archives of General Psychiatry 40:363–368, 1983

19. Martell DA, Dietz PE: Mentally disordered offenders who push or attempt to push victims onto subway tracks in New York City. Archives of General Psychiatry 49:472–475, 1992

20. Rabkin J: Criminal behavior of discharged mental patients: a critical appraisal of the research. Psychological Bulletin 86:1–27, 1979

21. Klassen D, O'Connor W: Assessing the risk of violence in released mental patients: a cross-validation study. Psychological Assessment: A Journal of Consulting and Clinical Psychology 1: 75–81, 1990

22. Monahan J: Mental disorder and violent behavior. American Psychologist 47:511–521, 1992

23. Shore D, Filson CR, Rae DS: Violent crime arrest rates of White House case subjects and matched control subjects. American Journal of Psychiatry 147: 746–750, 1990

24. Lindquist P, Allebeck P: Schizophrenia and crime: a longitudinal follow-up of 644 schizophrenics in Stockholm. British Journal of Psychiatry 157:345–350, 1990

25. Shah SA: Violence and the mentally ill. Journal of the California Alliance for the Mentally Ill 2:20–21, 1990

26. Bartels J, Drake RE, Wallach MA, et al: Characteristic hostility in schizophrenic outpatients. Schizophrenia Bulletin 17: 163–171, 1991

27. Link BG, Andrews H, Cullen FT: The violent and illegal behavior of mental patients reconsidered. American Sociological Review 57:275–292, 1992

28. Wesseley SC, Castle D, Douglas AJ, et al: The criminal careers of incident cases of schizophrenia. Psychological Medicine, in press

29. Psychiatrist killed by patient. American Medical News, Aug 16, 1985, p 17

30. Doctor stabbed by patient. Lafayette Advertiser, Apr 10, 1993, p A2

31. Dillon S: Social workers: targets in a violent society. New York Times, Nov 18, 1992, pp A1,B6

32. Steinwachs DM, Kasper JD, Skinner EA: Family Perspectives on Meeting the Needs for Care of Severely Mentally Ill Relatives: A National Survey. Arlington, Va, National Alliance for the Mentally Ill, 1992

33. Hatfield AB: Family Education in Mental Illness. New York, Guilford, 1990, p 33, citing a study by Swan RW, Lavitt MR: Patterns of Adjustment to Violence in Families of the Mentally Ill. New Orleans, Elizabeth Wisna Research Center, Tulane University School of Social Work, 1986

34. Straznickas KA, McNeil DE, Binder RL: Violence toward family caregivers by mentally ill relatives. Hospital and Community Psychiatry 44:385–387, 1993

35. Tardiff K: Characteristics of assaultive patients in private hospitals. American Journal of Psychiatry 141:1232–1235, 1984

36. Runions J, Prudo R: Problem behaviors encountered by families living with a schizophrenic member. Canadian Journal of Psychiatry 28:383–386, 1983

37. Acker J, Fine MJ: Families under siege: a mental health crisis. Philadelphia Inquirer, Sept 10–14 (5 parts), 1989, pp 1A–10A

38. Richardson D: Dangerousness and forgiveness. Journal of the California Alliance for the Mentally Ill 2:4–5, 1990

39. Phillips BJ: No one to ease his demon grip. Philadelphia Inquirer, July 23, 1991, p l7

40. Doe J: My brother might kill me. New York Times, May 6, 1987, p 13

41. Dearth N, Labenski BJ, Mott EM, et al: Families Helping Families: Living With Schizophrenia. New York, Norton, 1986

42. Swanson JW, Holzer CE, Ganju VK, et al: Violence and psychiatric disorder in the community: evidence from the Epidemiologic Catchment Area surveys. Hospital and Community Psychiatry 41:761–770, 1990

43. Hodgins S: Mental disorder, intellectual deficiency, and crime. Archives of General Psychiatry 49:476–483, 1992

44. Steadman HJ: Critically reassessing the accuracy of public perceptions of the dangerousness of the mentally ill. Journal of Health and Social Behavior 22:310–316, 1981

45. Yoder RM: The strange case of Howard Unruh. Saturday Evening Post, Sept 16, 1950, pp 24–25

46. Lunde DT, Morgan J: The Die Song. New York, Norton, 1980

47. Schreiber FR: The Shoemaker: The Anatomy of a Psychotic. New York, New American Library, 1983

48. Margolick D: Lowenstein killer moves toward freedom. New York Times, Nov 1, 1992, pp 49,54

49. Hinckley J, Hinckley JA: Breaking Points. Grand Rapids, Mich, Chosen Books, 1985

50. Pilot-test system assailed. Newsday, May 18, 1983, p 38

51. Tax lawyer's son committed. New York Times, May 9, 1983, p 15

52. Gorney C: Anatomy of a killer. Washington Post, Oct 11, 1984, pp B1,B6

53. Massacre at the mall. Washington Post, Nov 2, 1985, p A12

54. Sullivan R: Doctors had tried to hospitalize suspect in slashing on ferryboat. New York Times, Nov 11, 1986, pp Al,B3

55. Suspect's ills are described. Washington Post, Nov 29, 1987, p A20

56. Egginton J: Day of Fury. New York, William Morrow, 1991

57. Smothers R: Disturbed past of killer of 7 is unraveled. New York Times, Sept 16, 1989

58. Long K: James Brady: a life in search of himself. Atlanta Constitution, May 22, 1990, pp Al,A13

59. Furillo A: Why a killer was set free. San Francisco Examiner, July 14, 1991, pp Al,A10

60. Lyall S: Danger of mentally ill homeless to be re-evaluated in New York. New York Times, Jan 22, 1993, pp Al,B2

61. Bell C: Shooting suspect's bond is $250,000. Huntsville Times, Sept 5, l993, p B1

62. Anderson JW: Man smashes Constitution case. Washington Post, Oct 11, 1986, pp Al,B2

63. Maraniss D: The complete collector. Washington Post, Apr 1, 1990, pp Al,A23

64. Drifter indicted in church fires. Washington Post, Feb 14, 1992, p A19

65. Castenada R: Sen Glenn assaulted. Washington Post, Oct 26, 1989, p B1

66. Kattas A, Otis DB: A comparison of inpatients in an urban state hospital in 1975 and 1982. Hospital and Community Psychiatry 38:963–967, 1987

67. Marcus E: Man pleads guilty in deaths of father, stepmother. Washington Post, Feb 1, 1992, p B1

68. Woman who killed sons found insane. Washington Post, Feb 25, 1992, p C6

69. Duggan P: PG woman ruled insane in bike death. Washington Post, May 5, 1992, p D10

70. Man who said he killed parents may be sent to mental hospital. Washington Post, Aug 5, 1992, p D3

71. Jennings VT, Heath T: Gun that killed 4 was stolen in VA: suspect has history of violence, psychosis. Washington Post, Oct 14, 1992

72. Jennings VT: Family trouble plagued alleged Bethesda killer. Washington Post, Nov 15, 1992, p B1

73. Reiss AJ, Roth JA: Understanding and Preventing Violence. Washington, DC, National Academy Press, 1993, p 19

74. Petersson H, Gudjonsson GH: Psychiatric aspects of homicide. Acta Psychiatrica Scandinavica 64:363–372, 1981

75. Lagos JM, Perlmintter K, Saexinger H: Fear of the mentally ill: empirical support for the common man's response. American Journal of Psychiatry 134:1134–1137, 1977

76. Weiden PJ, Dixon L, Frances A, et al: Neuroleptic compliance in schizophrenia. Advances in Neuropsychiatry and Psychopharmacology, Vol 1: Schizophrenia Research. Edited by Tamminga C, Schulz C. New York, Raven, 1991

77. Smith LD: Medication refusal and the rehospitalized mentally ill inmate. Hospital and Community Psychiatry 40:491–496, 1989

78. Taylor P: Motives for offending amongst violent and psychotic men. British Journal of Psychiatry 147:491–498, 1985

79. Yesavage JA: Inpatient violence and the schizophrenic patient: an inverse correlation between danger-related events and neuroleptic levels. Biological Psychiatry 17:1331–1337, 1982

80. Weaver KE: Increasing the dose of antipsychotic medication to control violence (ltr). American Journal of Psychiatry 140:1274, 1983

81. Smith LD: Medication refusal and the rehospitalized mentally ill inmate. Hospital and Community Psychiatry 40:491–496, 1989

82. Baltimore man charged in mother's slaying. Washington Post, Dec 27, 1990, p D3

83. Crofton woman found guilty in mother's slaying. Washington Post, Sept 28, 1990, p D3

84. David A, Buchanan A, Reed A, et al: The assessment of insight in psychosis. British Journal of Psychiatry 161:599–602, 1992

85. Amador XF, Strauss DH: Poor insight in schizophrenia. Psychiatric Quarterly 64:305–319, 1993

86. Amador XF, Strauss DH, Yale SA, et al: Awareness of illness in schizophrenia. Schizophrenia Bulletin 17:113–132, 1991

87. Psychosis and civil rights. Wall Street Journal, Sept 28, 1990, p 15

88. Taylor PJ, Mullen P, Wessely S: Psychosis, violence, and crime, in Forensic Psychiatry: Clinical, Legal, and Ethical Issues. Edited by Gunn J, Taylor PJ. London, Butterworth & Heinemann, 1993

89. Krakowski MI, Convit A, Jaeger J, et al: Neurological impairment in violent schizophrenic inpatients. American Journal of Psychiatry 146:849–853, 1989

90. Apperson LJ, Mulvey EP, Lidz CW: Short-term clinical prediction of assaultive behavior: artifacts of research methods. American Journal of Psychiatry 150:1374–1379, 1993

91. Lidz CW, Mulvey EP, Gardner W: The accuracy of predictions of violence to others. JAMA 269:1007–1011, 1993

92. Monahan J, Steadman HJ: Toward a rejuvenation of risk assessment research, in Violence and Mental Disorder: Developments in Risk Assessment. Edited by Monahan J, Steadman H. Chicago, University of Chicago Press, 1994

93. Torrey EF: Nowhere to Go: The Tragic Odyssey of the Homeless Mentally Ill. New York, Harper and Row, 1988

94. Davidson R: A mental health crisis in Illinois. Chicago Tribune, Dec 9, 1991, p 18

95. Geller JL: A report on the "worst" state hospital recidivists in the US. Hospital and Community Psychiatry 43:904–908, 1992

96. Lafave HG, Pinkney AA, Gerber GJ: Criminal activity by psychiatric clients after hospital discharge. Hospital and Community Psychiatry 44:180–181, 1993

97. Navarro M: New York City to detain patients who fail to finish TB treatment. New York Times, Mar 10, 1993, pp 1,45

98. Lamb HR: Incompetency to stand trial: appropriateness and outcome. Archives of General Psychiatry 44:754–758, 1987

99. Bloom JD, Williams MH, Bigelow DA: Monitored conditional release of persons found not guilty by reason of insanity. American Journal of Psychiatry 148: 444–448, 1991

100. Ellard GA, Jenner PJ, Downs PA: An evaluation of the potential use of isioniazid, acetylisoniazid, and isonicotinic acid for monitoring the self-administration of drugs. British Journal of Clinical Pharmacology 10:369–381, 1980

101. Edelbrook PM, Zitman FG, Schreinder JN, et al: Amitriptyline metabolism in relation to antidepressant effect. Clinical Pharmacology and Therapeutics 35:467–473, 1984

Assessing the Evidence of a Link Between Mental Illness and Violence

Edward P. Mulvey, Ph.D.

The relationship of mental illness and violence is an issue of longstanding clinical and policy importance, and recent research on this association has sparked renewed debate. The author formulates six statements on the association that seem warranted by recent investigations and reviews the research evidence. In general, contrary to findings of earlier research, an association does appear to exist between mental illness and the likelihood of being involved in violent incidents. A dual diagnosis of mental illness and substance abuse probably significantly increases the risk for violence, and the association between mental illness and violence is probably significant even when demographic characteristics are taken into account. Given the considerable limitations of current research, priorities for future research include attention to the strength of the association for individual subjects, inclusion of adequate comparison groups of non-mentally-ill persons and a broad range of variables, and intensive studies of repetitively violent individuals over time.

Whether mentally ill persons are likely to commit violent acts in the community is an enduring, central issue in mental health law. Evidence about the strength of mental illness as a risk factor for violence is a pivotal point in debate about the appropriate use of involuntary hospitalization (1). Moreover, the contours of the relationship of mental illness and community violence are critical to the design of newer, community-based efforts to control violence by the mentally ill.

For the last 15 years or so, it was generally accepted that mentally ill individuals are no more likely than other people to commit violent acts in the community. Although clinical reports clearly documented that some people act violently on the basis of irrational beliefs or while in states of heightened symptomatology (2,3), reviews of the literature about violence by the mentally ill as a group showed no strong or consistent effect linking mental illness per se to community violence (4,5). Recently, however, new epidemiological studies have raised questions about whether the presence of mental illness appreciably raises the risk of an individual's being violent (6–9). In addition, two influential reviews (10,11) have come to the conclusion that mental disorder may, in the words of one of the authors, "be a robust and significant risk factor for the occurrence of violence" (11).

Because the question of the relationship of mental disorder to community violence is central to discussions about commitment policy and community services for mentally ill individuals, it is important to consider exactly what the present research does show. A careful consideration of what appears to be known and what issues are yet unresolved is a key step toward informed debate and research.

This paper formulates several statements about the relationship between mental illness and violent behavior in the community that seem warranted by recent investigations and reviews, and it examines the research evidence for them. Drawing on these discussions, it also presents several directions that should be pursued in future research.

What existing research does and does not show

On the basis of current research, six statements about the relationship between mental illness and violence can be made.

When this paper was published **Dr. Mulvey** *was associate professor of child psychiatry in the law and psychiatry program at the Western Psychiatric Institute and Clinic of the University of Pittsburgh School of Medicine, Pittsburgh, Pennsylvania. From the July 1994 issue of* Hospital and Community Psychiatry *(volume 45, pages 663–668).*

Mental illness appears to be a risk factor for violence in the community. A body of research, taken as a whole, supports the idea that an association exists between mental illness and violence in the general population. The amount and type of community violence that co-occur with particular disorders have been examined in clinical samples. About 20 percent of individuals appearing in psychiatric emergency rooms have been found to have some history of violent behavior (12). Higher overall levels of violent arrests have been noted for individuals with antisocial personality and substance abuse disorders (13) and with paranoid schizophrenia (14).

Recent studies that have followed samples of individuals released from mental hospitals have found more arrests for violent crimes in this group than in community samples (4,15–17). Moreover, several studies based on discharged hospital patients' self-reports of violent behavior have found higher levels of violence than expected (18–20), although the lack of comparison groups makes interpretation of the rates impossible. The level of violence found in samples of disordered individuals in the community varies widely, from 8 percent to about 45 percent, depending on the definitions of disorder and violence used.

The level of disorder seen in individuals with documented histories of violence has also been examined. Two of the most methodologically sophisticated studies have found a disproportionate number of disordered individuals in samples of incarcerated violent offenders (21,22). Schizophrenia and affective disorders were several times more prevalent in these samples than in the general population, even when age and race were statistically controlled for.

Two recent studies have examined epidemiological data sets to determine whether a relationship between mental disorder and violence exists. In a series of analyses using data from the National Institute of Mental Health's Epidemiologic Catchment Area surveys, Swanson and his colleagues (6,7) demonstrated that having a major mental illness, substance abuse only, or a mental disorder and substance abuse combined were each significantly related to a report of violence in the last year, even when covariation for demographic variables and history of institutional involvement were controlled for.

Similarly, Link and his colleagues (8,9), analyzing data from a project using the Psychiatric Epidemiology Research Interview (23), found higher rates of violence (measured by both self-reports and arrests) in a sample of mental patients than in residents from the same community in New York City who had never received psychiatric treatment. The effect held even when a range of variables that might have produced an artifactual relationship between psychiatric status and violence were controlled for.

Finally, in another recent investigation Mulvey and associates reproduced the findings of Swanson and Link and their colleagues, using different measures of symptomatology and violence and a different sampling strategy (Mulvey EP, Gardner WP, Lidz CW, Symptomatology and violence among mental patients, unpublished study, 1993). Data on symptoms, measured using the Brief Symptom Inventory (24), and on violence, measured using self-reports and collateral reports and official data, were collected in a three-wave panel design over a six-month follow-up period for 812 individuals with a mental disorder. A general measure of symptom severity over the six-month period was positively associated with the likelihood of a violent incident. In addition, a prospective test of whether symptomatology at the first interview could predict the occurrence of violence by the second or third interview was also positive, even when the subject's age, socioeconomic status, and history of violence were statistically controlled for.

Examined together, these studies make a convincing preliminary case for an association between mental illness and community violence. Each investigation suffers from some methodological shortcoming—for example, lack of clarity about the definition of mental illness, use of only official records, inadequacy of the comparison group, and problems of retrospective reporting—but the consistency of the findings is clear. As Monahan (11) concluded, the convergence of findings using a variety of samples and diverse measures in the studies above makes the denial of such an association difficult.

The size of the association between mental illness and violence, while statistically significant, does not appear to be very large. Also, the absolute risk for violence posed by mental illness is small. The correlations between reported symptoms and violence in the epidemiological studies (6–9) and Mulvey and associates' investigation were only in the .20 range. Other investigations of the power of mental illness alone as a predictor of violence have shown conflicting results and have been sensitive to the methodologies employed. This demonstration of a less than overwhelming association indicates considerable variability among individuals in the role that mental illness might play in relation to violence.

In addition, any association between mental illness and risk for violence must be interpreted in terms of relative risk and absolute risk. The studies to date have shown an increased relative risk for violence among individuals with mental illness compared with the general population; mental illness increases the likelihood of having a violent incident. However, important accompanying findings are that the absolute risk of violence among the mentally ill as a group is still very small and that only a small proportion of the violence in

> *The absolute risk of violence among the mentally ill population is very small, and only a small proportion of the violence in our society can be attributed to persons who are mentally ill.*

our society can be attributed to persons who are mentally ill (6).

The combination of a serious mental illness and a substance abuse disorder probably significantly increases the risk of involvement in a violent act. Investigations of levels of violence in various diagnostic groups and epidemiological studies point to a markedly increased risk for dually diagnosed individuals. This increased risk was also found in the study by Mulvey and associates using more comprehensive measures of violence.

In addition, findings from sociological investigations of the effect of alcohol use on violence indicate that long-term drinking patterns are more predictive of violence than is immediate use of alcohol in a situation (25,26). Although the mechanisms are not clear, an established pattern of alcohol or drug abuse appears to have a strong, although not necessarily interactive, effect with mental disorder to increase risk.

The association between mental illness and violence is probably significant even when demographic characteristics are taken into account. However, no sizable body of evidence clearly indicates the relative strength of mental illness as a risk factor for violence compared with other characteristics such as socioeconomic status or history of violence.

The recent investigations cited above show a significant association between mental illness and violence even after subjects' basic demographic characteristics are controlled for statistically. These independent results from large samples with a wide range of background characteristics provide considerable support for the position that the relationship between mental illness and violence is not simply an artifact in which the mental illness variable is serving as a proxy for other characteristics of the individual.

Previously, researchers such as Monahan and Steadman (27) were generally unable to find an association after these variables were controlled for. This lack of association could have resulted from the use of official records, in the vast majority of earlier studies, to determine incidence of violence. In these records, violence could have been more highly associated with demographic characteristics than it was in later studies based on self-reports of violence. As a result, the amount of variance to be explained by mental illness may have been greatly reduced, thus making the association difficult to find.

Although the level of violence among mental patients may be higher than previously thought, there is inadequate information about the levels of violence in matched comparison groups to make definitive statements about the relative power of mental illness as a risk factor compared with other subject characteristics. The few studies carried out with representative samples of comparison subjects have not used extensive measures of violence, which limits confidence in their estimates of the relative influence of variables. A comprehensive study of the levels and types of violence in samples of nondisordered individuals matched with samples of individuals with mental illness has not yet been done.

Active symptoms are probably more important as a risk factor than is simply the presence of an identifiable disorder. As would be expected, when the relationship of mental illness and violence has been examined using very broadly defined measures of these two constructs, the investigations have produced conflicting results.

In many studies, the presence of mental illness is determined by the involvement of the subject with the mental health system, thus confounding the ideas of "patient status" and "presence of an active mental disorder." Also, subjects at different points of involvement with the mental health system and at different stages of illness have all been represented under the rubric of "mentally ill." Violence, meanwhile, is often defined as an official report of an arrest or a recommitment for a violent incident, giving a filtered view of the level and types of incidents. This lack of clean definitions contributes to the variability of effect sizes observed.

Studies that have used self-reports of symptoms and violence or structured inventories for determining the presence of a mental disorder have proven somewhat more consistent and informative (6–9,28; Mulvey and associates, unpublished study, 1993). The pattern of their findings points to the importance of active symptomatology rather than simply to the presence of a mental disorder as a risk factor for violence. In Link and Stueve's study (9) in particular, controlling for reported symptoms eliminated the influence of patient status. Both the patient and the nontreated groups were more likely to have a violent incident when they also reported higher levels of active symptomatology. The association of mental illness and violence is probably best thought of as a dynamic process in which people are at increased risk at different times, possibly as the result of the emergence of particular types of symptoms or beliefs.

No clear information about the causal paths that produce the association between mental illness and violence is available. The literature to date has demonstrated an association between these two variables without a clear indication of causality between them. The presence of mental illness might be the first link in a chain of events resulting in violence. It is also possible that frequent violent encounters exacerbate a disorder.

Alternatively, these phenomena could simply coexist. Researchers in developmental psychopathology posit overlapping pathways to violent criminality and mental disorder (29), suggesting that violence and mental disorder are part of a larger constellation of maladaptive outcomes rather than links in a clearly causal chain of events. The data needed to test these possibilities are not available.

Directions for research

This set of statements points toward several future research directions. Obviously, recent investigations have forced a rethinking of the standard claim of "no relationship" between mental disorder and violent behavior in the community. At the same time, extant data provide only indirect guidance for policymaking and clinical interventions. Investigations of a different sort than those undertaken to date are necessary if we are to find out exactly what to make of this apparent association, both theoretically and practically.

A first step in making practical sense of the association between mental illness and community violence is to move beyond assessment of this relationship based simply on the size of the correlation coefficient generated. A statistically significant correlation does not necessarily validate the logic of particular clinical or legal policies. Similarly, a weak association does not imply that a focus on symptoms as a strategy for management of violence by mentally ill individuals is futile.

A closer look at the numbers that generate an association can often provide alternative ways to think critically about the usefulness of particular foci for interventions (30). Rather than thinking of the relationship of mental illness and violence as either "strong" or "weak" based on a single figure, it is important to look at the form of this relationship.

Data from the study by Mulvey and associates illustrate how a low measure of association between symptomatology and probability of violence does not necessarily show that symptomatology is irrelevant to the management of violence. In Figure 1, the bar graph shows the distribution of the scores from the measure of symptomatology, the global severity index from the Brief Symptom Inventory (24), in the sample of 812 mentally disordered individuals. Although patients showed a wide range of symptoms, their scores, as shown in the figure, fell in a narrow, and low, range of severity. The distribution of symptomatology scores is clearly skewed toward the low end, and this skewness may attenuate the size of the association between symptoms and violence in relation to a hypothetical sample with equal numbers of patients at each level of symptomatology.

The curve above the bar graph is the rate of violence for each level of symptomatology, calculated using an estimation procedure based on these data (31). This curve shows a mildly nonlinear relationship between the level of general symptomatology and the likelihood of a violent act occurring. The figure illustrates that although the correlation of symptoms

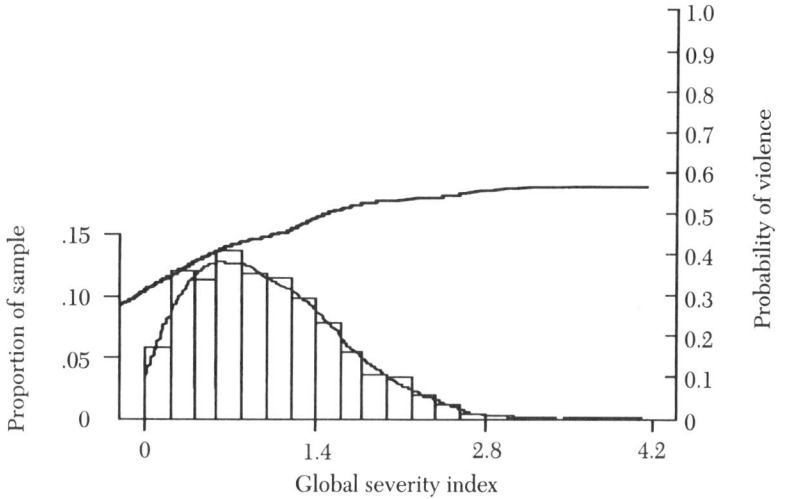

Figure 1

Distribution of general symptomatology[1] of 812 mentally ill individuals and the relationship of symptoms to probability of violence[2] at six-month follow-up

[1] Based on the global severity index of the Brief Symptom Inventory, scored from 0 to 4, with higher scores indicating greater symptomatology
[2] Probability of violence, represented by the line above the bar graph, is the proportion of people at that level of symptomatology who are violent.

and likelihood of violence is rather low, a number of individuals are highly symptomatic and substantially more likely than others to be violent.

An example of such an individual would be a man whose symptomatology takes the form of a delusional preoccupation with his wife's supposed infidelity, resulting in his violently confronting her. For him, the association of symptomatology and violence is strong, but these cases are rather rare in the overall sample.

The general point is that an overall coefficient of association describes only the linear trends in a total data set. It does not describe the strength of the association for every individual in the sample, nor does it allow for an adequate representation of the prevalence of individuals in a sample for whom the relationship is strong enough to warrant intervention or policy concern. Only by teasing apart the associations into more refined presentations like this one will we generate further fruitful discussions of the likely effects of intervention. Examination and comparison of the forms of the relationships between such factors as level of alcohol use, drug use, or prior history of violence would also be instructive.

A second clear step for future research would be to mount a systematic study of violence using an adequate comparison group of community residents who are not mentally ill. One central policy question is whether mental illness raises a person's risk of violence enough to warrant special treatment under the law. This question will remain unanswerable until more systematic studies of violence are undertaken with demographically similar subgroups of identified mentally ill individuals, individuals who are mentally ill but not identified as such, and community residents who are not mentally ill. More attempts to draw comparable subgroups are needed if we are to disentangle the effect of being identified as mentally ill by the mental health system from that of being mentally ill per se.

The range of variables examined in such studies should be broad, going well beyond simple documentation of mental illness, treatment history, and violence. Link and Stueve's intriguing findings (9) about the importance of symptoms related to personal control indicate that consideration should also be given to psychological belief systems that might be easily confused with mental illness or that might be explored only with those classified as mentally ill. Basic psychological traits, such as impulsivity, and the effects of social networks should also be considered.

In addition, it would be desirable to obtain careful specification of the types of violence documented to see if different types of violent incidents are more likely to occur in samples of mentally ill individuals, regardless of the overall level of violence found in the different groups (32). Finally, aspects of the patient's social environment or psychological functioning that might serve as protective factors against violence could be investigated.

Such a comprehensive approach to comparative studies of mentally ill and non-mentally-ill individuals is necessary if we are to provide convincing answers about the relative power of mental illness as a risk factor for violence, what might be different or the same about violence involving the mentally ill, and what policy approaches might be useful to address this issue.

A third step for researchers would be to develop specific theories about the mechanisms linking mental illness and violence. As mentioned earlier, the lack of theoretical clarity in this area is striking. Documentation of the prevalence of at least three types of cases would be helpful as an initial step: cases in which an individual feels compelled to act on his or her delusions, cases in which the onset of symptoms creates a stressor for others in the social environment and thus increases the likelihood of confrontation, and cases in which the disorientation of an illness decreases the likelihood of violence by limiting the individual's ability or energy to plan and focus actions.

It may well be that mental illness does not consistently increase the likelihood of violence within an individual, or that the mechanism by which it does increase risk varies over time. Knowing the variability in processes both within and across individuals would be valuable information for planning interventions and assessing their success. No doubt further systematic attention to theoretical development in this area could produce richer and more useful frameworks to guide comparison-group designs.

Some of the most valuable informa-

A variety of studies using very different approaches support the presence of a relationship between mental illness and violent behavior. However, the current state of the research provides very few leads about exactly what should be made of this association.

tion about the relationship between mental illness and violence would probably be obtained from intensive studies of repetitively violent individuals over time. The ultimate question for clinical and legal intervention is whether monitoring and intervention in relation to particular behaviors or life situations will reduce the likelihood of violence in the immediate future. The key to effective programming will lie in choosing the right points for intervention with the right types of individuals.

Deciding where to focus interventions, however, is more complicated than simply finding out what situational features surround violence by mentally ill persons. Knowing what situational factors, such as drinking, are present during violent incidents supplies only part of the picture. The regularity with which an individual engages in that particular behavior or enters that situation must also be known.

Consideration of drinking as a precipitant to violence provides an example. If an individual is involved in a violent incident every week and is drunk during 80 percent of his violent incidents, it would be tempting to assume that controlling drinking would have a large effect on the occurrence of violence. However, if the subject drinks heavily every day, the likelihood that alcohol is a highly influential factor in the violence might be questioned. Obviously, the subject is drunk six days of the week on which violence does not occur.

This example illustrates that definitive findings about the wisdom of focusing interventions on certain behaviors or social conditions to prevent violence can be obtained only by closely following the behavior of individuals over time. Knowledge of intrasubject variability on both violence and the conditions of interest is necessary to address the issue of causality.

The strategy for doing this kind of research would be to intensively follow a small group of potentially violent individuals over an extended period. Examining the fluctuations in the presence or absence of particular conditions and incidents of violence, using some variant of sequential analysis, would give the most telling information about factors worth targeting for intervention in that subgroup of individuals. Studies of this sort do not presently exist but would obviously be valuable for programming.

Conclusions
The former view that no significant relationship exists between mental illness and violent behavior in the community no longer seems tenable. Findings across a variety of studies using very different approaches support the presence of a relationship. However, the current state of the research provides very few leads about exactly what should be made of this association. We lack tested theoretical propositions about how mental illness and violence might be related, and we have little solid information about the actual magnitude of the association.

The challenge that lies ahead is one of further specifying the form of the relationship of mental illness and community violence and testing theories of how this relationship can differ across subgroups of mentally ill persons. Uncovering a broad relationship does not in itself promote sounder policy or more effective services. However, continued integration of research and service provision sensitive to what this relationship means in the lives of people with mental illness could move us toward this goal. ◆

Acknowledgments

Preparation of this paper was partly supported by funding from the violence and traumatic stress branch of the National Institute of Mental Health (grant MH-40030-08) and the U.S. Secret Service. The author thanks Charles W. Lidz, Ph.D., and William Gardner, Ph.D., for many of the ideas presented here and Jeffrey W. Swanson, Ph.D., for his critique of an earlier version.

References

1. Morse S: A preference for liberty: the case against involuntary commitment of the mentally disordered. California Law Review 70:54–106, 1982
2. Taylor P: Schizophrenia and violence, in Abnormal Offenders, Delinquency, and the Criminal Justice System. Edited by Gunn J, Farrington D. Chichester, England, Wiley, 1982
3. Wessely S, Taylor P: Madness and crime: criminology versus psychiatry. Criminal Justice and Mental Health 1:193–228, 1991
4. Rabkin JG: Criminal behavior of discharged mental patients: a critical appraisal of the literature. Psychological Bulletin 86:1–27, 1979
5. Mulvey EP, Blumstein A, Cohen J: Reframing the research question of mental patient criminality. International Journal of Law and Psychiatry 9:57–65, 1986
6. Swanson JW, Holzer CE, Ganju VK, et al: Violence and psychiatric disorder in the community: evidence from the Epidemiologic Catchment Area surveys. Hospital and Community Psychiatry 41:761–770, 1990
7. Swanson J: Mental disorder, substance abuse, and community violence, in Violence and Mental Disorders: Developments in Risk Assessment. Edited by Monahan J, Steadman HJ. Chicago, University of Chicago Press, 1994
8. Link BG, Andrews H, Cullen FT: Reconsidering the violent and illegal behavior of mental patients. American Sociological Review 57:275–292, 1992
9. Link BG, Stueve GA: Psychotic symptoms and the violent/illegal behavior of mental patients compared to community controls, in Violence and Mental Disorders: Developments in Risk Assessment. Edited by Monahan J, Steadman HJ. Chicago, University of Chicago Press, 1994
10. Otto R: The prediction of dangerous behavior: a review and analysis of "second generation" research. Forensic Reports 5:103–133, 1992
11. Monahan J: Mental disorder and violence behavior: perceptions and evidence. American Psychologist 47:511–521, 1992
12. Tardiff K, Sweillam A: Assault, suicide, and mental illness. Archives of General Psychiatry 37:164–169, 1980
13. Mulvey EP, Lidz CW: Clinical considerations in the prediction of dangerousness in mental patients. Clinical Psychology Review 4:379–401, 1984
14. Krakowski MI, Volavka J: Schizophrenic violence and psychopathology, in Current Approaches to the Prediction of Violence. Edited by Brizer DA, Crawner ML. Washington, DC, American Psychiatric Press, 1989
15. Giovannoni J, Gurel L: Socially disruptive behavior of ex-mental patients. Archives of General Psychiatry 17:146–153, 1967
16. Durbin J, Pasework R, Albers D: Criminality and mental illness: a study of arrest rates in a rural state. American Journal of Psychiatry 134:80–83, 1977
17. Schuerman LA, Kobrin S: Exposure of community health clients to the criminal justice system, in Mental Health and Criminal Justice. Edited by Teplin LA. Beverly Hills, Calif, Sage, 1984
18. Klassen D, O'Connor W: Assessing the risk of violence in released mental patients: a cross-validation study. Psychological Assessment: A Journal of Consulting and Clinical Psychology 1:75–81, 1990
19. Lidz CW, Mulvey EP, Gardner WP: The accuracy of predictions of violence to others. JAMA 269:1007–1011, 1993
20. Steadman H, Monahan J, Appelbaum P, et al: The MacArthur Risk Assessment Study, in Violence and Mental Disorder: Developments in Risk Assessment. Edited by Monahan J, Steadman HJ. Chicago, University of Chicago Press, 1994
21. Teplin L: The prevalence of severe mental disorder among urban jail detainees: comparison with the Epidemiologic Catchment Area Program. American Journal of Public Health 80:663–669, 1990
22. Current Description, Evaluation, and Recommendations for Treatment of Mentally Disordered Criminal Offenders. Sacramento, California Department of Corrections, Office of Health Care Services, 1989
23. Dohrenwend BP, Shrout P, Egri G, et al: Nonspecific psychological distress and other dimensions of psychopathology: measure for use in the general population. Archives of General Psychiatry 37:1229–1236, 1980
24. Derogatis LR, Melisaratos N: The Brief Symptom Inventory: an introductory report. Psychological Medicine 13:595–605, 1983
25. Reiss A, Roth J: Understanding and Preventing Violence. Washington, DC, National Academy Press, 1993
26. Fagan J: Intoxication and aggression, in Drugs and Crime. Edited by Tonry M, Wilson JG. Chicago, University of Chicago Press, 1990
27. Monahan J, Steadman H: Crime and mental disorder: an epidemiological approach, in Crime and Justice: An Annual Review of Research. Edited by Tonry M, Morris N. Chicago, University of Chicago Press, 1983
28. Steadman HJ, Felson RR: Self reports of violence: ex-mental patients and the general population. Criminology 22:321–342, 1984
29. Robin L, Rutter M (eds): Straight and Devious Pathways From Childhood to Adulthood. Cambridge, England, Cambridge University Press, 1990
30. Rosenthal R: How are we doing in soft psychology? American Psychologist 45:775–776, 1990
31. Cleveland WS: Robust locally weighted regression and smoothing scatterplots. Journal of the American Statistical Association 74:829–836, 1979
32. Mulvey EP, Lidz CW: Measuring patient violence in dangerousness research. Law and Human Behavior 17:277–288, 1993

Violence and Psychiatric Disorder in the Community: Evidence From Epidemiologic Catchment Area Surveys

Jeffrey W. Swanson, Ph.D.
Charles E. Holzer III, Ph.D.
Vijay K. Ganju, Ph.D.
Robert Tsutomu Jono, M.S.P.H.

The link between mental disorder and violent behavior is a subject of paramount importance to the fields of psychiatry and public mental health policy. Yet despite a voluminous research literature, basic questions persist: To what extent do psychiatric disorders increase the risk of assaultive behavior, if at all? Are people in the community with untreated mental illness and those seen in clinical settings equally prone toward violence? What are the relative probabilities of violence associated with substance abuse, other specific psychiatric disorders, and dual diagnoses? Is the connection between mental illness and violence largely conditioned by other variables such as socioeconomic status?

We address the above questions using data from three communities surveyed in the National Institute of Mental Health's Epidemiologic Catchment Area project, which is the largest community study of psychiatric disorders ever conducted in the United States.

Background

In a 1984 review of the literature, Mullen (1) concluded that mental abnormality by itself contributes little to

Data from the Epidemiologic Catchment Area survey were used to examine the relationship between violence and psychiatric disorders among adults living in the community. Psychiatric assessment of survey respondents was based on the Diagnostic Interview Schedule, which also provided self-report information about violent behavior. Those who reported violent behavior within the preceding year tended to be young, male, and of low socioeconomic status, and more than half met DSM-III criteria for one or more psychiatric disorders. Subjects with alcohol or drug use disorders were more than twice as likely as those with schizophrenia to report violent behavior. In a multivariate model controlling for demographic covariates and substance abuse, the occurrence of major mental illness was associated with a threefold increase in the odds of violent behavior. The risk of violence increased with co-occurring alcohol or other drug use disorders and with the number of diagnoses for which respondents met DSM-III criteria.

the prediction of violent behavior. He suggested that there are subgroups of mentally abnormal individuals at higher and others at lower risk for violence.

Nevertheless, Mullen lamented, "The literature is largely inadequate to delineate such ... risk groups with the degree of certainty ideally needed to instruct clinical decisions." More recently, Mills (2) discussed the thorny issues surrounding the psychi-

---

When this paper was published Dr. Swanson was assistant professor and Dr. Holzer was associate professor in the department of psychiatry and behavioral sciences at the University of Texas Medical Branch at Galveston. Dr. Ganju was director of special programs with the office of strategic planning in the Texas Department of Mental Health and Mental Retardation in Austin. Mr. Jono was a research associate in the Center for Cross-Cultural Research at the University of Texas Medical Branch at Galveston. From the July 1990 issue of Hospital and Community Psychiatry *(volume 41, pages 761–770). Revised to incorporate corrections described in "Violence and ECA Data" (letter to editor), September 1991 (volume 42, pages 954–955).*

atric assessment of dangerousness among the mentally ill, and after reviewing current studies concluded, "The authors' findings may have little to do with the overall pool of the mentally ill, to the extent that those who present or who are seen in psychiatric evaluation settings are 'preselected.' More comprehensive conclusions must await a study [of dangerousness] that examines the entire population of the significantly mentally ill."

Although questions posed at the public policy level may appear straightforward ("Do the mentally ill pose a danger in the community?"), answers developed in clinical settings are more complex and ambiguous. Different kinds of illnesses contribute to violence by means of unique etiologic pathways. People with the same diagnosis behave differently under different conditions depending on their age and gender, living environment, personal history, cultural orientation, and position in the social structure.

It is even difficult to define violence and mental illness as independent terms. For a number of psychiatric disorders described in *DSM-III-R*, violent behavior is virtually an essential diagnostic feature; they include antisocial personality disorder, borderline personality disorder, intermittent explosive disorder, and sexual sadism. Diagnostic survey data cannot really address the question of whether such disorders cause violence, since assaultive behavior lies at the core of what is labeled as psychiatric disorder. For a number of other diagnoses, notably schizophrenia, bipolar disorder, and substance abuse, *DSM-III-R* lists violent behavior as an associated feature; although it is not a necessary symptom, violent behavior increases the likelihood that these diagnoses will be given (3,4).

A large number of studies have been conducted on violent behavior among psychiatric patients (5–13). Across this body of research, estimates of the prevalence of violence range widely, based on different time intervals, case mixes, periods in the patient's career, and criteria for assessing violence. For example, Petrie and associates (6) examined admission records at a state psychiatric hospital and counted the number of patients for whom a threat of assaultive behavior was listed as a presenting symptom on admission. They found violence indicated in 62.6 percent of the cases—not surprisingly a high percentage, since "danger to others or self" is a chief criterion for admission and for civil commitment to state hospitals.

Estimates of the prevalence of violence range widely, based on different time intervals, case mixes, periods in the patient's career, and criteria for assessing violence.

Contrast the Petrie study of violence preceding hospitalization with Tardiff and Sweillam's study (7) of violence in the hospital. The authors reviewed records of long-stay psychiatric inpatients and counted actual assaults committed in the hospital. Using this criterion, they found the three-month prevalence of violence to be 7 percent—not surprisingly a lower percentage than in the Petrie study, since many patients become less violent once they are in the therapeutic milieu of a hospital. In fact, many of the nonviolent hospital patients might have been termed dangerous before admission, as Tardiff and Sweillam have shown elsewhere (13).

Regarding the question of which diagnoses are most strongly associated with assaultive behavior, the bias of hospital- and clinic-based studies becomes apparent. Krakowski and associates (3) reviewed 13 studies of psychiatric diagnoses among violent patients and reported that "schizophrenics as a group tend to be more violent than patients with other diagnoses." Indeed, schizophrenia is a common diagnosis of mental hospital patients deemed to be violent. However, this finding does not tell us whether persons with schizophrenia who reside in the community are more violence-prone than anyone else, since those who are violent may be found more often in the hospital.

Krakowski and associates (3) further reported that patients with major affective disorder, including manic-depressive illness, have a lower propensity toward violence than patients with other kinds of psychopathology. Although persons with manic disorder often engage in threatening behavior, according to these researchers, "The . . . irritability and hostility noted in manics does not usually progress to actual violent behavior." But once again, as they point out, this finding cannot be generalized to all people with manic disorder; it may be an artifact of the clinical selection process and of the rapid response to treatment observed in manic patients.

Another body of research has assessed psychopathology among violent criminals (14–21). As with research on psychiatric patients, it is difficult to draw a comprehensive picture of violence and mental illness from these diverse studies. One study examines substance abuse among homicide perpetrators, another looks at personality disorders in a general group of prisoners, and still another considers the criminally insane as a special population.

In the area of public policy and the law, a sizable literature exists surrounding issues of civil commitment of the mentally ill pursuant to their dangerousness (22–24). These studies constitute a vigorous debate about the success (and failure) of psychiatrists in predicting clinically whether a patient will engage in violent behavior if released or if not committed (25–29). The lack of consensus belies the paucity of sound empirical data on which such predictions can reliably be made.

All of these studies illustrate the importance of the relationship between violence and psychiatric disorder. However, they tell us little about this phenomenon as it occurs among people not already labeled by the mental health service system, the criminal justice system, or both. The NIMH Epidemiologic Catchment Area (ECA) project avoided this shortcoming by focusing its assessment on community residents randomly selected.

The ECA data

The data in this study are drawn from three of the five large surveys that made up the NIMH ECA project. Representative sample surveys of adult household resident populations were carried out in New Haven, Baltimore, St. Louis, Raleigh-Durham, and Los Angeles (30,31). Structured diagnostic interviews were conducted between 1980 and 1983 with 3,000 to 5,000 household residents at each site. Eaton (32) and Holzer (33) and their associates have reported the details of the ECA sampling design. Myers (34) and Burnam (35) and their associates have reported prevalence rates for the individual sites.

For this analysis, the data from Baltimore, Raleigh-Durham, and Los Angeles were pooled to form one large data base of approximately 10,000 respondents. The New Haven and St. Louis surveys were excluded for reasons explained below. The data were weighted based on respondents' probabilities of selection.

Because samples were drawn in several stages of selection (tracts, households, residents), the pooled data provide a sampling variance that is somewhat larger than would have occurred in a simple random sample. Average design effects for the analysis presented herein range from 1.4 to 1.8. (See Holzer and associates [33, 36] for a detailed discussion of ECA sample weighting and issues surrounding analysis of the pooled data.)

Measurement

Psychiatric disorder

The core of the interview at all five sites was the Diagnostic Interview Schedule (DIS) (37). The DIS is a structured interview designed for use by trained lay persons. The DIS generates *DSM-III* diagnoses for current-time intervals and lifetime. The diagnoses to be considered here include schizophrenia, major depression, mania or bipolar disorder, alcohol abuse or dependence, drug abuse or dependence, obsessive-compulsive disorder, panic disorder, and phobia.

The time interval chosen was one year; to count as a positive case, the respondent had to meet *DSM-III* criteria for a given disorder during the 12 months preceding the interview.

A respondent who met criteria for more than one disorder, for example, alcoholism and depression, was initially counted as a case in the statistics for each of those disorders. We also present data on respondents with multiple diagnoses compared with those with a single diagnosis.

Violence

The DIS items indicating violent behavior were contained in the diagnostic sections for antisocial personality disorder (items 1–4) and for alcohol abuse or dependence disorder (item 5). They include the following:

1. Did you ever hit or throw things at your wife/husband/partner? [If so] Were you ever the one who threw things first, regardless of who started the argument? Did you hit or throw things first on more than one occasion?

2. Have you every spanked or hit a child, (yours or anyone else's) hard enough so that he or she had bruises or had to stay in bed or see a doctor?

3. Since age 18, have you been in more than one fight that came to swapping blows, other than fights with your husband/wife/partner?

4. Have you ever used a weapon like a stick, knife, or gun in a fight since you were 18?

5. Have you ever gotten into physical fights while drinking?

Recency of the behaviors described in items 1–4 was established by a probe at the end of the diagnostic section for antisocial personality disorder: "When is the last time you did any of these things, such as [individual violence items mentioned]?" Recency for item 5 was assessed specifically for that item in the three ECA sites that were pooled for this analysis. Specific recency for item 5 was not assessed in the New Haven and St. Louis surveys.

Hence, "fights while drinking" that occurred long in the past could erroneously be included in the construct as operationalized for these sites. This is made evident by rates two to three times higher in these two surveys than in the others. For this reason, the New Haven and St. Louis sites were removed from the analysis.

In short, using a three-site pooled data base, we counted a respondent positive for violent behavior if he or she endorsed at least one of the items listed above and said that some such behavior occurred during the 12 months preceding the interview.

One other feature of the DIS posed a potential problem for analysis of the violence items in the Baltimore data. Originally, the DIS allowed some items to be skipped, including those related to violent behavior, if a respondent reported no misconduct during childhood or adolescence. Fortunately, two of the three sites that we used did not skip the questions in their interviews. Still, in the data from Baltimore, information is missing on items 1–4 if the respondent failed to report any childhood behaviors such as playing hooky from school, telling lies, getting into fights at school, or running away from home overnight.

We handled this problem by taking the population that did provide information on item 5 (getting in fights while drinking) and using it as the denominator for the Baltimore sample in the overall index. This approach had the effect of slightly lowering our estimate of the general prevalence of violence and may have introduced a bias. However, when we compared the adjusted Baltimore estimate with the rates from the other two sites that did not have missing data, we found that all three rates were virtually the same, that is, within a range of 1.6 percentage points, with Baltimore in the middle.

A more serious problem was that the ECA data provide no adequate quantitative measure of violence. Though the items are varied and cover a wide range of behavior, they overlap considerably and are not specific in terms of severity and frequency. We did count the number of positive items, but the count gives only a rough and indiscriminate indicator of the severity and frequency of violent behavior.

Logically speaking, a respondent who committed multiple acts of felonious assault (even homicide) cannot be distinguished from someone with only a single, less serious episode to report. This is hardly a trivial limitation; it prevents us from inferring the actual degree of dangerousness associated with specific disorders. All that we really have is a blunt measure of the presence or absence of any violent behavior in association with specific psychiatric diagnoses. Nevertheless, this rough measure provides some valuable information that was previously unavailable in a large-scale community survey.

As with the DIS diagnoses, we chose one year as the reference period for the violent behavior, though other periods were available in the data. We reasoned that one year is a reasonably long current-time interval, giving an adequate opportunity for violent behavior to be manifest when the propensity for it exists. Using a shorter interval would have produced lower rates and may have underestimated the true risk of violence. Going beyond one year, on the other hand, would have risked understatement of the problem due to inadequate recall.

Socioeconomic status
Socioeconomic status was measured by a ranking that combined information about the respondent's occupation status, educational level, and household income. Occupations were ranked according to mean percentiles on educational level and income for all incumbents to a given occupational title in the 1980 U.S. Census, following a procedure developed by Nam and Powers (38). That ranking was used to form a percentile score that was then averaged with the respondent's own education and income percentile scores. The result was an index from 0 to 100, with lower scores indicating lower socioeconomic status. The ECA respondents were then divided into four classes roughly corresponding to quartiles: 0–25, 26–50, 51–75, and 76–100 (36).

Methods of analysis
Frequency analyses were conducted to determine the prevalence and patterns of self-reported violence by age, sex, socioeconomic status, and diagnoses. Standard errors were calcul-

> *Being young, male, and of low socioeconomic status all were found to be associated with violent behavior. Race was not related to violence when socioeconomic status was controlled.*

ed for the rates of violence by diagnosis, using a statistical method for estimating sample variance in large surveys (39).

A multivariate model of the predictors of violent behavior was also developed. Logistic regression was used to analyze the entire pattern of rates of violence by gender, age, socioeconomic status, presence of substance abuse, presence of other major psychiatric diagnosis, and the interaction (cross-product) of substance abuse and mental disorder. This technique produced a measure of the fit between the observed rates in the ECA data and the values predicted by a relative risk model that was based on the relationships among these variables. The logistic regression analysis included tests for the statistical significance of each variable controlling for the others.

Results
One-year prevalence of violent behavior
The pooled data included 10,059 respondents on whom there was some information about violent behavior during the current year. Of these, 140 respondents (1.4 percent) reported getting in fights while drinking, 109 (1.1 percent) reported hitting a spouse or partner, 27 (.2 percent) reported hitting a child, 183 (1.8 percent) reported getting in physical fights with someone other than a partner, and 109 (1.1 percent) reported having used a weapon in a fight.

Of note is the low prevalence of child abuse relative to the other items; only .2 percent admitted hitting a child hard enough to cause bruises or require bed rest or medical attention. The comparatively low frequency of this item may result from the fact that subjects most likely to behave violently (young unmarried men) have little contact with children.

Although violence against children may actually be less common than other kinds of violence, some amount of underreporting is also likely due to the stigma surrounding child abuse and the fear of legal sanction. This highlights the larger issue of the reliability of self-report surveys as a method of assessing especially sensitive or illegal behaviors. While we cannot estimate the magnitude of underreporting bias affecting particular items, we can cite evidence for acceptable reliability and validity in the ECA data base as a whole (31).

Considering the five items assessing violent behavior together, 236 respondents (2.4 percent) reported positive responses on one item, while 132 (1.3 percent) reported positive responses on two or more items. Eight persons had positive responses on four of the five items, but none responded positively on all items. As an overall assessment of the prevalence of violent behavior, 368 respondents (3.7 percent) responded positively to at least one of the items for the one-year period preceding the interview. The prevalence rates and weighted sample sizes for the individual sites were Baltimore, 3.9 percent (N=3,102); Raleigh-Durham, 3.08 percent (N=3,845); and Los Angeles, 4.14 percent (N=3,113).

Sociodemographic relationships
Being young, male, and of low socioeconomic status all were found to be associated with violent behavior. Race was not related to violence when socioeconomic status was controlled. The rate of self-reported violence among males was more than twice as high as that among females, 5.29 percent compared with 2.21 percent. Of all respondents between 18 and 29 years old, 7.34 percent re-

Table 1

Percentage of respondents reporting violent behavior by sex, age, and socioeconomic status

Sex and age	Weighted N of respondents[1]	Socioeconomic status[2]			
		0–25	26–50	51–75	76–100
Male					
18 to 29	1,600	16.09	11.68	8.06	6.05
30 to 44	1,278	7.65	6.23	4.57	2.56
45 to 64	1,272	3.34	2.00	2.14	.29
65 and over	567	.20	.30	.00	.00
Female					
18 to 29	1,635	9.11	5.01	2.46	3.27
30 to 44	1,377	3.92	3.47	1.77	1.17
45 to 64	1,472	.93	.25	.54	1.01
65 and over	822	.00	.00	.00	.00

[1] Weighted Ns are rounded; percentages may not correspond to whole numbers.
[2] Scores based on occupation, education, and income ranking; lower scores indicate lower status.

ported violent behavior, while among those between the ages of 30 and 44 the rate dropped to 3.59 percent. Among those between the ages of 45 and 64, the rate was only 1.22 percent, and in the group over age 65, the prevalence of violence was less than 1 percent.

Low socioeconomic status also was found to be related to violent behavior, particularly among younger respondents. Table 1 presents rates of violent behavior by sex, age, and socioeconomic status. Among both males and females under age 45, rates of violence in the lowest socioeconomic group were about three times higher than in the highest socioeconomic group.

Prevalence of psychiatric disorder among those who report being violent

Of the 368 people who reported some violent behavior in the preceding year, more than half—55.5 percent—met criteria for a psychiatric disorder, compared with 19.6 percent of nonviolent respondents. Substance abuse was by far the most prevalent diagnosis among those who were violent; 41.64 percent had alcohol or drug abuse disorders, compared with only 4.93 percent of the nonviolent respondents.

The prevalence of affective disorder was three times higher among respondents who were violent (9.37 percent) than among those who were not (2.95 percent). The same was true for the prevalence of schizophrenia or schizophreniform disorder (3.92 percent versus 1.03 percent). The difference was less pronounced for the prevalence of anxiety disorders; the rate was 20.13 percent among the violent respondents, compared with 14.13 percent among those who were not violent.

Patterns of violence by diagnosis

Table 2 shows the prevalence of violent behavior reported by those with various psychiatric illnesses, initially considered without regard to multiple diagnoses. Each of the disorders was associated with some risk of violence; however, the risk was highest among those with alcohol abuse or dependence disorders (24.57 percent) and other drug abuse or dependence disorders (34.74 percent).

The specific findings of some previous research reports concerning diagnoses other than substance abuse were not confirmed in these community survey data. Contrary to a number of studies of patient populations, violence was not significantly more prevalent among persons with schizophrenia than among those with other disorders. Further, those with affective disorders, including manic depressive illness, did not have lower rates of assaultive behavior than those with other disorders. Indeed, with the exception of phobia, those with other mental disorders manifested remarkably similar rates of assaultive behavior, from 10.66 percent to 12.69 percent, across a range of diagnoses, from obsessive compulsive disorder to schizophrenia.

Table 3 shows rates of violent behavior by sex and diagnostic group. Males with a diagnosis of anxiety disorder had a higher rate of violence than did females with this disorder. However, among respondents with major mental disorder and with substance abuse, males and females did not significantly differ in their rates of violence.

When we take a closer look at the respondents who met *DSM-III* criteria for more than one disorder, a somewhat different picture emerges regarding violence. For example, violence was reported by a fair number of respondents with a DIS diagnosis

Table 2

Diagnostic Interview Schedule diagnoses of respondents reporting violent behavior in the last year

Diagnosis	Weighted N of respondents[1]	Percent violent	Standard error
No disorder	7,870	2.05	.0020
Phobia	1,323	4.97	.0077
Obsessive-compulsive disorder	182	10.66	.0303
Panic disorder	90	11.56	.0425
Major depression	282	11.68	.0224
Major depression with grief	308	10.70	.0210
Mania or bipolar disorder	30	11.02	.0582
Schizophrenia or schizophreniform disorder	114	12.69	.0319
Cannabis abuse or dependence	191	19.25	.0428
Alcohol abuse or dependence	586	24.57	.0225
Other drug abuse or dependence	99	34.74	.0651

[1] Column cannot be summed for total N because some respondents met criteria for more than one disorder.

of panic disorder. On the surface, this finding might be interpreted in light of the *DSM-III* criteria for panic disorder, which may include an intense fear of doing something uncontrolled during an anxiety attack.

However, of the 90 respondents with panic disorder, about two-thirds also met DIS/*DSM-III* criteria for affective disorders, substance abuse, or schizophrenia. These individuals were also more likely to report violent behavior. Therefore, it would be misleading to naively attribute a given rate of violence to panic disorder among these respondents.

DSM-III states that while panic attacks may occur in association with schizophrenia and major depression, the diagnosis of panic disorder should not be given if the attacks are due to these other disorders.

To address this issue of multiple diagnoses and violence, we created a typology of four diagnostic groups: anxiety disorder, affective disorder, substance abuse, and schizophrenia spectrum disorders. Combining these categories in all possible ways resulted in 16 types, all of which occurred empirically in the data base (for example, five respondents met criteria for a disorder in all four of our diagnostic groups). Table 4 presents rates of self-reported violence by diagnostic type.

Those with a diagnosis only in the anxiety category had rates of violence virtually identical to those with no disorder at all (2.37 percent and 2.05 percent, respectively). Those with a diagnosis only in the affective category showed just a slightly higher rate, with 3.45 percent reporting violent actions. Interestingly, however, when diagnoses of anxiety and affective disorders were combined, the rate of violence more than tripled to 11 percent. Clearly, dual diagnoses, with their higher levels of psychiatric symptomatology, accounted for the higher rates of violence observed among all those with anxiety and affective disorders.

Among those with schizophrenia or schizophreniform disorder alone, the relative risk of violence was substantial (8 percent versus 2 percent among those with no disorder), but the absolute prevalence was low. In other words, 92 percent of persons with a diagnosis of schizophrenia only in a community population were not violent by their own report. This finding appears to be at odds with some hospital-based portrayals of the violent tendencies of schizophrenic patients relative to those with other diagnoses. In combination with substance abuse or affective symptomatology, however, those with schizophrenia showed a higher propensity toward assaultiveness than those with a diagnosis of schizophrenia only.

To further examine the notion that having multiple disorders increases the risk of violence, we simply counted the actual number of diagnoses (without regard to the four diagnostic categories) for which each respondent met *DSM-III* criteria. We combined cannabis with other drug abuse as one disorder, and we collapsed the two categories of depression—major depression and grief—into one disorder irrespective of whether the illness was associated with bereavement. We then calculated rates of self-reported violent behavior for those with no diagnosis, one diagnosis, two diagnoses, and three or more diagnoses. The results are shown in Figure 1. There appears to be a nearly linear relationship between the number of diagnoses and the rate of violence; the rate triples as the number of diagnoses increases from one to three or more.

The finding of higher rates of violence with multiple diagnoses might be interpreted in several ways. One interpretation might be that number of diagnoses is really an indicator of the gross amount and variety of psy-

Table 3

Percentage of respondents reporting violent behavior in the last year, by sex and diagnostic group

Diagnostic group	Male			Female		
	N[1]	% violent	SE	N[1]	% violent	SE
No disorder	3,728	2.74	.0033	4,143	1.11	.0023
Anxiety disorders	484	8.87	.0147	960	3.25	.0070
Major affective disorder or schizophrenia	142	11.30	.0291	266	10.03	.0224
Alcohol or drug disorder	591	21.08	.0217	150	21.70	.0457

[1] Column cannot be summed for total N because some respondents met criteria for more than one disorder.

Figure 1

Percentage of respondents reporting violent behavior by number of diagnoses on the Diagnostic Interview Schedule

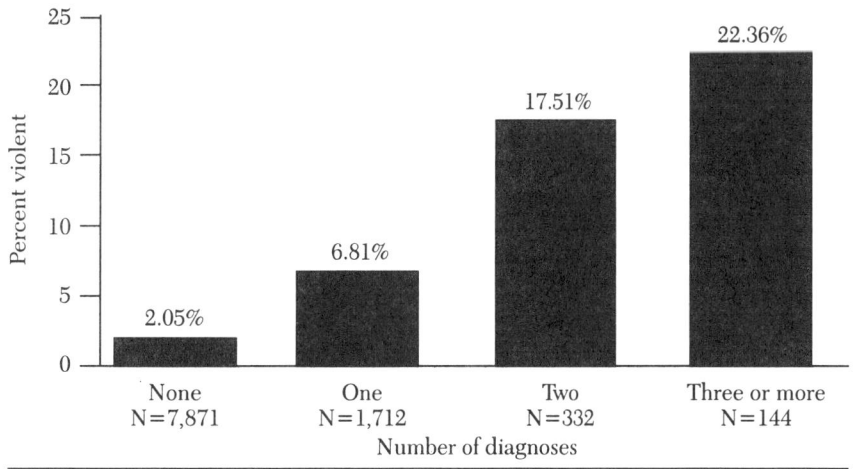

Table 4

Percentage of respondents reporting violent behavior, categorized by types of diagnoses on the Diagnostic Interview Schedule

Diagnostic group	Weighted N of respondents[1]	Percent violent
No disorder	8,066	2.05
One diagnostic group		
Anxiety disorder only	1,160	2.37
Affective disorder only	142	3.45
Schizophrenia only	26	8.36
Substance abuse only	533	21.30
Two diagnostic groups		
Schizophrenia and anxiety	36	4.29
Affective disorder and anxiety	99	11.09
Substance abuse and anxiety	119	20.25
Schizophrenia and affective disorder	10	21.09
Affective disorder and substance abuse	29	29.19
Schizophrenia and substance abuse	3	30.33
Three diagnostic groups		
Schizophrenia, substance abuse, and anxiety	23	15.22
Affective disorder, substance abuse, and anxiety	24	16.71
Schizophrenia, affective disorder, and anxiety	12	17.09
Schizophrenia, substance abuse, and affective disorder	1	100.00
Four diagnostic groups		
Schizophrenia, substance abuse, affective disorder, and anxiety	5	28.75

[1] Total N respondents=10,223

chopathology present; the more symptoms and problems someone has, the more likely that violent behavior will be among them (especially since the violence items are explicitly included in DIS/DSM-III symptomatology).

Another interpretation might suggest that people with multiple diagnoses are more likely to have a substance abuse disorder, of which violence itself is sometimes a symptom. A third interpretation might be that people who report many symptoms in different diagnostic sections of the DIS are "yea-sayers," and by that token are more likely to say yes to the violence questions as well. Probably each of these notions contains some truth.

Although we have no direct indicators of the frequency or severity of violent behavior, we did consider the number of positive items on the violence index. It could be argued that a respondent whose violent behavior has been frequent and severe would be more likely to respond positively to multiple items assessing violent behavior. However, this sort of interpretation requires caution because of overlap in the variables. Striking a spouse with an object while drinking may constitute a single recent episode, but it could result in a positive response to three of the five items. Nevertheless, counting the items may approximate severity and frequency at least roughly. Table 5 shows the results of that count.

Of the few people who reported violent behavior even though they had no psychiatric disorder, most reported positive responses on only one of the items. Among those who did have a DIS diagnosis and reported some violent action as well, about half responded positively to more than one item. Clearly there is a relationship between the rate of violence and the number of positive responses reported within the diagnostic groups. Except for two diagnoses (panic and mania), the prevalence of positive responses on multiple (three or more) items correlates perfectly with the rate of any violence. We infer from this finding that the diagnoses with the highest risk of any violence occurring are also those most associated with severe and frequent violence, for example, violence directed toward various victims, use of weapons, and so forth.

Table 6 shows the percentage of respondents who gave positive responses to the individual items concerning violence, by DIS diagnosis. For most of the disorders, we noted a fairly even distribution of responses across the items. Violence toward spouses or partners was reported with about equal frequency as violence toward others, while assaultive action against children was less commonly reported. An exception can be noted among those with alcohol and drug use disorders, who more often reported violence toward someone other than a spouse.

Another exception to the pattern of violence occurred among those with

Table 5

Percentage of respondents with one or more positive responses to Diagnostic Interview Schedule (DIS) items related to violent behavior, by DIS diagnosis

Diagnosis	Weighted N of respondents[1]	N positive responses		
		1	2	3+
No disorder	7,870	1.59	.35	.12
Phobia	1,323	2.38	1.23	1.37
Obsessive-compulsive disorder	182	5.92	2.01	2.73
Panic disorder	90	2.14	2.62	6.79
Major depression	282	6.03	2.61	3.05
Major depression with grief	308	5.52	2.39	2.79
Mania or bipolar disorder	30	8.96	2.07	.00
Schizophrenia or schizophreniform disorder	114	4.11	4.89	3.68
Cannabis abuse or dependence	191	11.69	3.17	4.38
Alcohol abuse or dependence	586	13.50	4.94	6.12
Other drug abuse or dependence	99	17.48	9.70	7.55

[1] Column cannot be summed for total N because some respondents met criteria for more than one disorder.

panic disorder. Seven percent of respondents, a relatively high proportion, responded positively to the child abuse item. However, as discussed earlier, most of the people with panic disorder actually met criteria for another psychiatric illness as well, such as affective disorder, substance abuse, or schizophrenia. This phenomenon was an artifact of the lack of exclusion rules in the DIS. Of those who had a diagnosis of DIS panic disorder only, none responded positively on the child abuse item.

Subjects with mania or bipolar disorder provided a final exception to the pattern. In particular, no one with mania reported hitting someone other than a spouse-partner or child, and no one with mania reported using a weapon in a fight. The absence of positive responses on some items could be expected among this group, however, since their overall prevalence is very low and the number of respondents with mania was very small (there were 30 in the three-site data base for whom current information on violence was available).

In general, as rates on the violence index increase from one diagnostic group to another, rates on the individual items follow accordingly. No one item accounts for a disproportionate number of positive responses overall, with the exception of "fights while drinking" for those with alcohol and drug abuse disorders. It might be argued that we should have excluded this item in our assessment of violence among alcoholics, since it was extracted from the DIS section for establishing the diagnosis of alcoholism in the first place.

It is true that for the diagnosis of alcoholism our measures are confounded to a minor extent. But we calculated that at least 75 percent of alcoholics in the ECA surveys met *DSM-III* criteria for their disorder without reporting that they got into fights while drinking. A comparable majority of alcoholics who were violent would have been classified as such on our violence index even if the item concerning fights while drinking had been excluded. In our opinion, had we excluded the item, it would have biased the index in the direction of underreporting. After all, a person who is violent while drinking is definitely violent, though he may not be an alcoholic by *DSM-III* rules.

Multivariate analysis

Logistic regression analysis was used to examine simultaneously the relative effects on violence of substance abuse, major mental illness, and selected sociodemographic variables. Variables were added one at a time stepwise and retained if they produced an effect that was significant at the $p<.01$ level. All the variables in the final model, shown in Table 7, were significant at each step. Initial models were run with epidemologic catchment area site and race (black, Hispanic, white, and other) included as predictors. Neither of these variables had significant main effects or interaction effects.

The final model is based on rates of violence across all combinations of the following categorical variables: sex, age group, socioeconomic status, major mental disorder only (schizo-

Table 6

Percentage of respondents with positive responses to violence-related items on the Diagnostic Interview Schedule (DIS), by DIS diagnosis

Diagnosis	Weighted N of respondents[1]	Percent of positive responses				
		Drinking, fighting	Hit partner	Hit child	Hit other	Weapon fight
No disorder	7,870	.45	.62	.14	.80	.40
Phobia	1,323	2.06	2.11	.43	2.48	2.09
Obsessive-compulsive disorder	182	3.88	5.50	.65	4.17	4.21
Panic disorder	90	4.05	5.91	7.02	7.35	6.73
Major depression	282	4.09	5.24	1.21	4.82	5.03
Major depression or grief	308	3.75	4.80	1.11	4.41	4.61
Mania or bipolar disorder	30	5.72	5.30	2.07	.00	.00
Schizophrenia	114	6.15	5.32	.75	6.94	8.58
Cannabis abuse or dependence	191	11.70	6.00	.53	7.18	6.28
Alcohol abuse or dependence	586	15.82	6.02	1.49	11.65	8.04
Other drug abuse or dependence	99	18.15	12.59	.00	15.47	14.33

[1] Column cannot be summed for total N because some respondents met criteria for more than one disorder.

Table 7

Logistic regression model of predictors of self-reported violent behavior in the past year[1]

Independent variable	Odds ratio	95% confidence intervals		Adjusted χ^2	$p<$[2]
		Lower	Upper		
Male	1.74	1.37	2.22	19.90	.001
Age	.40	.35	.47	145.78	.0001
Socioeconomic status	.74	.66	.84	21.33	.0001
Major mental disorder only	3.42	2.16	5.41	27.68	.0001
Substance abuse only	8.07	6.27	10.38	262.36	.0001
Major mental disorder and substance abuse	10.22	5.87	17.77	67.69	.0001

[1] Weighted N respondents= 10,024
[2] df = 1
Hosmer and Lemeshow goodness-of-fit statistic=7.13, df=8, p=.52
Model χ^2=883.45, df=6, p<.0001
Rank-order correlation coefficent of predicted to observed frequencies=.84

phrenia, bipolar disorder, or depression), substance abuse only (alcohol or other drug use disorder), and dual diagnosis (major mental disorder and substance abuse combined). Respondents with no disorder form the comparison group for the odds ratios attached to the diagnostic categories shown in the model.

Of the 128 possible cells resulting from the cross-tabulation of these variables, 112 actually occurred in the three-site ECA database with information on violence. All variables in the final model were statistically associated with violence at significance levels of $p<.001$ or better after adjusting for design effects. The adequacy of the model's overall fit is seen in the nonsignificance of the Hosmer and Lemeshow goodness-of-fit statistic (7.13, df=8, p=.52). The observed cell frequencies and the probabilities of violence predicted by this model were not significantly at variance, but were correlated by a rank-order coefficient of .84.

To summarize the information shown in Table 7, the model had an acceptable fit with these data. Being male, young, and of lower socioeconomic status were all associated with violent behavior. Controlling for these demographic variables, having a major mental disorder by itself significantly increased the odds of violence (odds ratio=3.42; predicted probability of violence=.07). Substance abuse disorder was associated with an even greater risk of violent behavior (odds ratio=8.0; predicted probability of violence=.20), as was the combination of mental disorder with alcohol or other drug use disorder (odds ratio=10.2; predicted probability of violence=.23).

Discussion

The ECA data clearly demonstrate that individuals in the community with psychiatric disorders are more likely to engage in assaultive behavior, by their own report, than those who are free of mental illness and substance abuse. Considered separately, without regard for multiple diagnoses, each disorder that we examined was associated with increased risk of violence. However, persons with anxiety disorder only (those who did not meet criteria for affective disorder, substance abuse, or schizophrenia in addition) had about the same rate of violence as those with no disorder (2.4 percent). Those with affective disorder only also had a relatively low rate of violence (3.4 percent).

In contrast, alcohol and drug abuse and the presence of more than one diagnosis increased the risk of violence substantially. Respondents with disorders associated with higher levels of assaultiveness (especially substance abuse) were also more likely to respond positively to multiple items on the violence index; that is, there was a greater chance that they had assaulted more than one kind of victim and that they had used a weapon. In general, it appears that the group of substance abusers not only includes the highest percentage of violent individuals; those individuals also commit more severe acts of violence with greater frequency. However, given the limitations of our data, we cannot be certain about this conclusion.

Another important finding of this study concerns the social and personal context within which both psychopathology and violent behavior are embedded. Specifically, in our data the effect of psychiatric disorders on assaultiveness varied not only by what kind and how many diagnoses someone had, but by who manifested these conditions: being male, young, and of lower socioeconomic status increased the risk substantially, apart from psychiatric illness.

These data may dispel certain myths about the dangerousness of people with particular forms of mental illness, most notably schizophrenia. It would seem that public fear of persons with schizophrenia living in the community is largely unwarranted, though not totally groundless: 12.7 percent of all those with schizophrenia in this study reported violent behavior during the year. Among those with only schizophrenia or schizophreniform disorder (those who did not also meet criteria for substance abuse or affective or anxiety disorders), the violence rate was lower, 8.4 percent, though still several times higher than among those with no disorder. Even so, citizens stand a much greater chance of being assaulted by an alcoholic: 25 percent of those with alcoholism were violent by their own report.

Significantly, there are far greater numbers of alcohol abusers in the community than there are persons with schizophrenia, and alcohol abusers are considerably less likely to receive treatment. Moreover, a proportion of the harmful acts committed by persons with schizophrenia may be influenced by drug and alcohol use as well: nearly a third of those with schizophrenia or schizophreniform disorder in this study also met criteria for alcohol or drug abuse or dependence.

We have shown that the interaction between substance abuse and major psychopathology is a statistically significant predictor of violence.

Previous studies of violent behavior and mental illness in patient populations have not been representative of people in the community with the same disorders. In particular, clinic-based studies may systematically overestimate violence among persons with schizophrenia while underestimating violence associated with major affective disorder. Indeed, rates of violence among those with schizophrenia, affective disorders, and anxiety disorders appear to be remarkably similar, in the range of 11 percent to 13 percent, when people with multiple diagnoses are included as cases for each of their disorders.

With the strong trend toward short-term hospital stay and community-based care for the seriously mentally ill, it is important to know as precisely as possible the risks that those with specific psychiatric disorders and personal characteristics may or may not pose to others. The ECA surveys represent a major step forward in understanding the complex linkages between mental health and violence in the community. ♦

Acknowledgments

The data analysis for this paper was supported in part by a National Institute of Mental Health contract to Dr. Swanson. The Epidemiologic Catchment Area Program was supported in part by NIMH grants MH–34224 and MH–15783. A fuller analysis of these data is presented in

Swanson JW: Mental disorder, substance abuse, and community violence: an epidemiological approach, in Violence and Mental Disorder. Edited by Monahan J, Steadman H. Chicago, University of Chicago Press, 1994

References

1. Mullen PE: Mental disorder and dangerousness. Australian and New Zealand Journal of Psychiatry 18:8–17, 1984

2. Mills MJ: Civil commitment: the relationship between perceived dangerousness and mental illness. Archives of General Psychiatry 45:770–772, 1988

3. Krakowski M, Volavka J, Brizer D: Psychopathology and violence: a review of literature. Comprehensive Psychiatry 27:131–148, 1986

4. Burrowes KL, Hales RE, Arrington E: Research on the biologic aspects of violence. Psychiatric Clinics of North America 11:499–509, 1988

5. Krakowski M, Jaeger J, Volavka J: Violence and psychopathology: a longitudinal study. Comprehensive Psychiatry 29:174–181, 1988

6. Petrie WM, Lauson EC, Hollander MH: Violence in geriatric patients. JAMA 248:443–444, 1982

7. Tardiff K, Sweillam A: Assaultive behavior among chronic inpatients. American Journal of Psychiatry 139:212–215, 1982

8. Craig TJ: An epidemiological study of problems associated with violence among psychiatric inpatients. American Journal of Psychiatry 139:1262–1266, 1982

9. Myers KM, Dunner DL: Self- and other-directed violence on a closed acute-care ward. Psychiatric Quarterly 56:178–188, 1984

10. Herman JL: Histories of violence in an outpatient population: an exploratory study. American Journal of Orthopsychiatry 56:137–141, 1986

11. Holcomb WR, Ahr PR: Arrest rates among young adult psychiatric patients treated in inpatient and outparient settings. Hospital and Community Psychiatry 39:52–57, 1988

12. Sosowsky L: Crime and violence among mental patients reconsidered in view of the new legal relationships between the state and the mentally ill. American Journal of Psychiatry 135.33–42, 1978

13. Tardiff K, Sweillam A: Assault, suicide, and mental illness. Archives of General Psychiatry 37:164–169, 1980

14. Hafner H, Boker W: Crimes of Violence by Mentally Abnormal Offenders. Translated by Marshall H. Cambridge, England, Cambridge University Press, 1982

15. Taylor PJ, Parrot JM: Elderly offenders: a study of age-related factors among custodially remanded prisoners. British Journal of Psychiatry 152:340–346, 1988

16. Ormstad K, Karlsson T, Enkler L, et al: Patterns in sharp force fatalities: a comprehensive forensic medical study. Journal of the Forensic Sciences 31:529–542, 1986

17. Tardiff K: Patterns and major determinants of homicide in the United States. Hospital and Community Psychiatry 36:632–639, 1985

18. Harruff RC, Francisco JT, Elkins SK, et al: Cocaine and homicide in Memphis and Shelby County: an epidemic of violence. Journal of Forensic Sciences 33:1231–1237, 1988

19. Welte JW, Miller BA: Alcohol use by violent and property offenders. Journal of Drug and Alcohol Dependence 19:313–324, 1987

20. Senay EC, Wettstein R: Drugs and homicide: a theory. Journal of Drug and Alcohol Dependence 12:157–166, 1983

21. Steadman HJ, Cocozza JJ: Careers of the Criminally Insane. Lexington, Mass, Lexington, 1974

22. Webster CD, Ben-Aron MH, Hucker SJ: Dangerousness: Probability and Prediction, Psychiatry and Public Policy. Cambridge, England, Cambridge University Press, 1985

23. Miller RD: Outpatient civil commitment of the mentally ill: an overview and an update. Behavioral Science and Law 6:99–118, 1988

24. Brooks AD:Outpatient commitment for the chronically mentally ill: law and policy. New Directions for Mental Health Services, no 36:117–128, 1987

25. Segal SP, Watson MA, Goldfinger SM, et al: Civil commitment in the psychiatric emergency room, 1: the assessment of dangerousness by emergency room clinicians. Archives of General Psychiatry 45:749–752, 1988

26. Cocozza JJ, Steadman HJ: The failure of psychiatric prediction of dangerousness. clear and convincing evidence. Rutgers Law Review 29:1048–1101, 1976

27. Megaree E: The prediction of violent behaviour. Criminal Justice and Behaviour 3:3–21, 1976

28. Greenland C: Psychiatry and the prediction of dangerousness. Journal of Psychiatric Treatment and Evaluation 2:97–103, 1980

29. Monahan J: The Clinical Prediction of Violent Behavior. Rockville, Md, National Institute of Mental Health, 1981

30. Regier DA, Myers JK, Kramer M, et al: The Epidemiologic Catchment Area Program. Archives of General Psychiatry 41:934–941, 1984

31. Eaton WW, Kessler LG (eds): Epidemiological Field Methods in Psychiatry: The NIMH Epidemiologic Catchment Area Study. New York, Academic Press, 1985

32. Eaton WW, Holzer CE, Von Korff M, et al: The design of the Epidemiologic Catchment Area surveys. Archives of General Psychiatry 41:942–948, 1984

33. Holzer CE, Spitznagel E, Jordan KB, et al: Sampling the household population, in Epidemiologic Field Methods in Psychiatry. Edited by Eaton WW, Kessler LG. New York, Academic Press, 1985

34. Myers JK, Weissman MM, Tischler CE, et al: Six months' prevalence of psychiatric disorders in three communities. Archives of General Psychiatry 41:959–967, 1984

35. Burnam MA, Hough RL, Escobar JI, et al: Six months' prevalence of specific psychiatric disorders among Mexican Americans and non-Hispanic whites in Los Angeles. Archives of General Psychiatry 44:687–694, 1987

36. Holzer CE, Shea BM, Swanson JW, et al: The increased risk for specific psychiatric disorders among persons of low socioeconomic status: evidence from the NIMH Epidemiologic Catchment Area study. American Journal of Social Psychiatry 6:259–271, 1986

37. Robins LN, Helzer JE, Croughan J, et al: National Institute of Mental Health Diagnostic Interview Schedule: its history, characteristics, and validity. Archives of General Psychiatry 38:381–389, 1981

38. Nam CB, Powers MG: The Socioeconomic Approach to Status Measurement. Houston, Cap & Gown Press, 1983

39. Shah BV: SESUDAAN: Standard Errors Program for Computing of Standard Rates From Sample Survey Data: Research Triangle Park, NC, Research Triangle Institute, 1981

Clinical Symptoms, Neurological Impairment, and Prediction of Violence in Psychiatric Inpatients

Menahem I. Krakowski, M.D., Ph.D.
Pal Czobor, Ph.D.

As Monahan (1) has pointed out, it is important to understand the specific features of mental disorder that carry increased risk for violence by psychiatric patients. In exploring these specific features, the literature has often focused on a single set of variables, such as psychiatric symptoms on hospital admission, that are assessed at a single time point. Emphasis has been on contrasting violent patients with nonviolent patients and treating all violent patients as a homogeneous group. A more differentiated clinical picture is presented here, one that considers the independent underlying deficits that contribute to violence and the type of violence (transient or persistent).

The psychiatric literature has emphasized the importance of neurological impairment in the genesis of violence (2,3). Psychotic symptoms also play an important role (4,5). In acutely psychotic patients, scores on items of the Brief Psychiatric Rating Scale (BPRS) (6) indicating conceptual disorganization, hallucinations, and unusual thought content were positively correlated with subsequent rate of violence (7–9). A strong positive association was found between psychotic symptoms, as measured by the Psychotic Symptomatology Scale, and recent violent behavior (10).

Violence, in the aforementioned literature, has been linked either to neu-

Objective: The study sought to identify basic clinical symptoms of violent inpatients and to determine the relationship between these symptoms and two outcome measures: whether violence was persistent or transient, and length of stay on a secure care unit designed to control violent behavior. *Methods:* Thirty-eight patients consecutively admitted to the secure care unit were assessed using a quantified neurological scale, the Brief Psychiatric Rating Scale, and a modified version of the Social Participation Rating Scale, which measured participation in unit activities. Because there was considerable overlap among these clinical measures, factor analysis was applied to isolate underlying clinical factors. *Results:* Factor analysis consistently identified two independent factors at different time points. The first factor, which consisted of various psychiatric symptoms and behavioral abnormalities, was indicative of general impairment. The second factor was bipolar, reflecting a positive association with neurological impairment and a negative association with paranoid symptoms. A differential association between these two factors and the outcome variables was found. Length of stay, a measure of perceived dangerousness, was best predicted by the general impairment factor, whereas persistent violence was predicted primarily by the bipolar factor. *Conclusions:* The data confirmed an association between persistent violence and neurological impairment. The study underscores the need for differential treatment of violent behavior in psychiatric inpatients, as different psychopathological processes might be involved.

rological impairment or to psychiatric symptoms. It should be noted, however, that several studies have shown an association between these two types of variables; neurological signs were

found to be positively correlated with thought disorder and other psychotic symptoms (11,12). Clinical experience indicates that ward behaviors, which are also of interest here, are influenced

---

When this paper was published **Dr. Krakowski** *was a research psychiatrist at the Nathan S. Kline Institute for Psychiatric Research in Orangeburg, New York, and assistant professor of psychiatry at New York University Medical Center in New York City.* **Dr. Czobor** *was a research scientist at the Nathan S. Kline Institute. From the July 1994 issue of* Hospital and Community Psychiatry *(volume 45, pages 700–705).*

both by psychiatric symptoms and by neurological impairment. Given the multiple interconnections between these variables, we must identify the underlying deficits in terms that effectively describe the patient's manifest clinical impairment and symptoms.

The violent behavior itself must be analyzed further. On the basis of the literature and some of our previous findings described below, it seems particularly important to distinguish between transient violence and persistent violence, as these two forms may be related to different clinical variables. A positive association exists between paranoid symptoms and transient violence. Patients with such symptoms are often reported to be violent when acutely ill, that is, before admission to the hospital or early in the course of hospitalization. However, their symptoms remit quickly, and therefore they account for less violence later in their stay than various other patients, such as those with prominent psychotic disorganization, diagnoses of undifferentiated schizophrenia, or organic mental syndrome (13,14). Neurological impairment, on the other hand, shows a strong positive association with persistent violence; a disproportionate percentage of violent repetitive offenders evidence some sort of brain dysfunction (15–18).

In line with these considerations, in previous studies we proposed a typology of violence based on state and trait factors (19,20). We contrasted transient violence with persistent violence; transient violence was hypothesized to be associated with acute decompensation and prominent paranoid symptoms, and persistent violence to be associated with neurological impairment.

One of the studies, conducted with a much larger sample than the study reported here, dealt primarily with the issue of whether neurological impairment contributed to violent behavior by inpatients on a secure care unit specifically designed to control violence (19). The study reported here, done on the same secure unit, is also based on the persistent or transient model of violent behavior. However, the clinical variables have been expanded to include psychiatric symptoms and ward behaviors as well as neurological impairment. These clinical variables were examined in relation to an additional outcome measure besides violence: length of stay on the unit.

In this study, underlying deficits based on measures of clinical symptoms are identified through factor analysis and are used for the prediction of persistent violence. Because all the patients in this study presented with histories of violence, what is of interest here is the persistence of violence on an inpatient unit designed to control such behavior.

Length of stay on the unit was chosen as an outcome measure because it reflected clinicians' overall impression of the patient's dangerousness; patients returned to their home wards when clinicians judged them to be sufficiently improved. It is of practical importance to find out how this major outcome variable is related to basic clinical symptoms.

Methods
Setting and subjects
The seven-month study was conducted on a 15-bed secure care unit designed for the management of violent behavior. The unit is located in a 1,300-bed state psychiatric facility serving predominantly indigent inner-city patients in a large metropolitan area. Control of violent behavior on the unit is achieved by various means, including a high staff-patient ratio, a better-trained staff, and close monitoring of all behaviors. Patients are never allowed off the unit, and there is no opportunity for any substance abuse. The mean±SD length of stay is 54.5±26.5 days. At the end of their stay, patients are transferred back to their home wards. Discharge decisions are made by two unit psychiatrists in consultation with unit staff.

The study subjects consisted of 38 inpatients consecutively admitted to the unit from November 1984 to May 1985. Many subjects in this group were also part of a larger study of the relationship between neurological impairment and violent behavior (19).

All the patients had been physically assaultive on their home wards and were transferred to the secure care unit to bring their violent behavior under control. Twenty-six of the patients were male. Eight were white, and 30 were nonwhite. Their mean± SD age was 29.3±7.6 years.

Diagnoses for all patients were established by consensus of two psychiatrists using *DSM-III-R* criteria. Twenty-three patients had a diagnosis of schizophrenia; two, bipolar disorder; six, personality disorder; and seven, mental retardation. In the group with mental retardation, psychotic features consistent with schizophrenia were also present. This condition is usually viewed as a superimposition of a schizophrenic illness on preexisting mental retardation (21,22).

Information on the patients' history of substance abuse and arrests for violent crimes was obtained from patient records and interviews because of its possible relevance to violent behavior. Eighteen, or 47 percent, of the 38 patients had a history of substance abuse. Eight of these patients had a history of both alcohol and drug abuse, six of alcohol abuse alone, and four of drug abuse alone. Nineteen patients, or 50 percent, had been arrested for some crime, and 13 of the 19 had been arrested for a violent crime. Information was also obtained on all medications administered to the patients while on the secure care unit.

Clinical assessment instruments
Patients were assessed using three instruments: a quantified neurological scale (23), the Brief Psychiatric Rating Scale (BPRS) (6), and a modified version of the Social Participation Rating Scale (24).

The quantified neurological scale assessed cerebellar, cortical, and cranial nerve abnormalities as well as soft signs. The 56 items included Romberg's sign, hopping, finger-to-nose, pronation and supination, heel-to-shin, extraocular movements, facial asymmetry, hearing, gag reflex, tongue asymmetry, muscle strength asymmetry, finger-thumb opposition, foot taps, tendon reflexes asymmetry, stereognosis, graphesthesia, face-hand test, and inconsistency of handedness. The scale was administered by two physicians with formal training in neurology. Interrater reliability was measured with 32 patients; the intraclass correlation coefficient for the total neurological score was .91.

The 18-item Brief Psychiatric Rating Scale was used to evaluate the patients' psychiatric symptoms. BPRS evaluations were made by two raters; one rated all the patients weekly, and the other rated all patients intermittently. Interrater reliability was established at the outset of the study; the intraclass correlation coefficient was .93. Factor analysis involving all 18 BPRS items yielded five factors reflecting symptoms in the areas of anxiety-depression, anergia, thought disturbance, activation, and hostility-suspiciousness (25).

A modified form of the Social Participation Rating Scale (SPRS) was used to assess the degree of participation and appropriateness of patients' behavior in four major activities on the ward: group discussions, recreational activities, calisthenics, and morning grooming activity. These ratings were included because little is known about the overall functioning of violent patients in routine ward activities. Two activity therapists rated each activity on a 5-point scale, with higher scores indicating increasing dysfunction. One activity therapist made weekly ratings of all patients for the duration of the study; the other rated the patients for five weeks. The intraclass correlation coefficient for the two raters was .91.

The data analyses used the total score on the quantified neurological scale, the total SPRS score, and BPRS factor scores on anergia, thought disturbance, activation, and hostility-suspiciousness.

Outcome measures
A patient's outcome was measured by two variables: the nature of the violent behavior (recidivistic or persistent violence versus transient violence) and the patient's length of stay on the unit. Length of stay was chosen as an outcome measure because it reflected clinicians' perceptions of the patient's level of dangerousness.

Recidivistic or persistent violence was defined as two or more assaults during the patient's stay on the unit; transient violence was defined as only one incident or no incident after transfer to the unit. Violent behavior was defined as physical assaults (physically aggressive acts), verbal assaults (verbal threats of bodily harm) directed at another patient or a staff member, and assaults against property. Verbal and property assaults were included because they were found to be positively related to physical assaults (Pearson's $r=.61$, $p=.0001$ for verbal assaults; $r=.41$, $p=.01$ for assaults against property). All assaults occurring on the unit were carefully recorded and differentiated from other disruptive behaviors such as agitation and uncooperativeness.

Procedures and statistical analyses
The study's main hypothesis was that manifest clinical variables, such as psychiatric symptoms, ward behaviors, and neurological impairment, can best be understood in the context of more basic underlying deficits that determine further occurrence of violence and length of stay. This hypothesis was examined using data gathered in the first, third, and last weeks of stay. The third week was selected because all patients stayed on the unit a sufficient time for at least three weekly assessments.

In line with the above hypothesis, there were two steps in the analyses. The first required the identification of underlying factors. Because our clinical variables were interrelated, a few underlying factors could explain most of their variation. Factor analysis (principal component analysis with unrotated factors) was used to identify the most important underlying factors.

The second step was to examine the relationship of the underlying variables to the outcome variables of persistent or transient violence and length of stay. Multiple regression analysis was used to examine length of stay, and logistic regression analysis was used to examine type of violence, a dichotomous variable.

All 38 patients had been physically assaultive before their transfer to the secure care unit, but they showed a varying degree of assaultiveness while on the unit. Twenty-five patients were involved in two or more incidents of assault, while 13 were involved in only a single incident that occurred shortly after transfer or were not involved in any incident. Thus the distribution was markedly skewed, with a mean±SD of 7.66±9.92 incidents. There were no differences in the ratio of physical to verbal or property assaults among the different diagnostic groups.

The average number of neurological abnormalities among the patients was 5.38. No distinct pattern of abnormal neurological findings implicated a single brain area, hemisphere, or functional system. Several regions or systems were involved; soft signs, cerebellar abnormalities, and cortical signs were found.

Patients with a history of substance abuse did not differ from the other patients in the number of physical, verbal, or property assaults or in neurological impairment, length of stay on the unit, or paranoid or psychotic symptoms.

Factor analysis yielded two main factors that accounted for most of the variance consistently at all three time points. Factor 1, which was indicative of general impairment, accounted for 47 percent, 50 percent, and 52 percent of the variance for the first, third, and last weeks of stay. Factor 2, indicative of specific impairment, accounted for 22 percent, 17 percent, and 17 percent of the variance during those periods.

Results for all scales with high factor loadings (.50 or more) are presented in Table 1. The loadings indicate that the different scales made similar contributions to the factors at all three time points.

Factor 1 had consistently high loadings on all clinical measures with the exception of hostility-suspiciousness and neurological impairment. For factor 2, only neurological impairment and hostility-suspiciousness had high factor loadings at all three time points. But while neurological impairment had a positive loading, hostility-suspiciousness had a negative loading. Factor 2, then, was bipolar.

To what extent did these two factors predict persistence of violence and length of stay? Factor 2, the bipolar factor, was related to persistence of violence at all three time points (N=38, slope=1.44, $\chi^2=6.48$, df=2, p=.01 for the first week; N=38, slope=1.34, $\chi^2=5.10$, df=2, p=.02 for the third week; N=38, slope=1.25, $\chi^2=4.33$, df=2, p=.04 for the last week). Factor

1, the general factor, was not related to persistence of violence in the total group of subjects at any time point.

Interestingly, the opposite was true for length of stay; factor 1 was related to length of stay at all three time points (slope=8.24, t=2.03, df=36, p=.049 for the first week; slope=11.36, t=2.78, df=36, p=.01 for the third week; slope=13, t=3.4, df=36, p=.002 for the last week). Factor 2 was significantly related to length of stay only for the first week (slope=9.1, t=2.24, df=36, p=.05).

To check whether the inclusion of nonpsychotic patients influenced these results, we repeated all the above analyses after excluding the six patients with personality disorders. The results were essentially unchanged, with one exception: when patients with personality disorders were excluded, factor 1 made a significant contribution to persistence of violence during the last week of stay (N=38; slope=−1.14; χ^2=3.84, df=2, p=.05).

More detailed analyses were performed to improve understanding of how individual clinical measures were related to persistence of violence. An analysis of variance showed that patients who were repeatedly violent had more severe neurological impairment than those who were not severely impaired (F=4.65, df=1,37, p=.04). Patients who were transiently violent evidenced more paranoid symptoms, especially during their first week on the unit (F=6.56, df=1,36, p=.015). These differences were consistent with the factor loadings for factor 2 described above.

To better understand how the individual clinical measures were related to length of stay, post hoc Pearson's correlations were performed. Psychiatric symptoms and ward behaviors, as assessed during the third and last weeks, determined length of stay. There was a positive correlation between length of stay and total BPRS score and total SPRS score for the third week (BPRS, N=38, r=.37, p=.02; SPRS, N=38, r=.44, p=.01) as well as for the last week (BPRS, N=38, r=.49, p=.002; SPRS, N=38, r=.49, p=.002), but not for the first week. Length of stay, however, was not related to neurological impairment nor to the number of physical, verbal, or property assaults occurring over a fixed period.

We did some additional post hoc tests to check for possible confounding factors. Comparisons of patients who were persistently violent and transiently violent revealed no difference in level of neuroleptic dosage (as measured in chlorpromazine equivalents) or in incidence of substance abuse. These factors, then, could not account for the difference in neurological impairment.

Table 1

Factor analysis[1] of clinical variables contributing to persistent or transient violence and to length of stay on a unit for control of violent behavior

Variable	Factor 1			Factor 2		
	Week 1	Week 3	Last week	Week 1	Week 3	Last week
Social Participation Rating Scale total score	.73	.70	.79	—	—	—
Brief Psychiatric Rating Scale factor						
Anergia	.85	.83	.86	—	—	—
Thought disturbance	.86	.80	.72	—	—	—
Activation	.71	.73	.73	—	—	—
Hostility-suspiciousness	—[2]	.62	.57	−.84	−.58	−.59
Neurological impairment total score	—	—	.65	.61	.79	.54

[1] Principal component method with no rotation
[2] Factor loading below .50

Discussion

In earlier studies we proposed a model in which transient violence was associated with acute decompensation, whereas persistent violence was associated with subtle neurological impairment (19,20). This study explores this model through a systematic assessment of psychiatric symptomatology, ward behaviors, and neurological impairment in violent inpatients admitted to a unit specially designed to control violent behavior.

The patients' psychiatric symptoms, ward behaviors, and neurological impairment can best be understood in terms of more basic underlying factors. Two basic factors were identified independently and consistently at three different time points. The first factor was indicative of general impairment; it consisted of various psychiatric symptoms and behavioral abnormalities, except for neurological dysfunction and paranoid symptoms, which formed a separate and more specific factor. The latter was bipolar in nature, with neurological impairment contributing positively and paranoid symptoms contributing negatively.

This bipolar factor, organic impairment versus paranoia, is suggestive of the flexibility of illness, or the capability of symptoms to remit over time. It calls to mind certain distinctions drawn in the literature between reversible and irreversible aspects of psychotic illnesses, such as organic versus functional (26) or process versus reactive (27). Neurological impairment corresponds to the organic or process component, and hostility-suspiciousness (as it appears within this factor) to the reactive or functional dimension.

This finding is consistent with reports in the literature that symptoms associated with structural changes in the brain do not respond well to treatment, in contrast to paranoid delusions and hallucinations (28), and may be associated with a more severe illness, including premorbid asociality (29). Paranoid symptoms have also been contrasted with cognitive impairment in schizophrenia (30). The association between reversibility of illness and paranoid symptoms is also consistent with reports of better outcomes for paranoid schizophrenia (31,32).

Persistence of violence was predicted by factor 2, which encompassed neurologic impairment and hostility-suspiciousness. This factor represents the reversibility or irreversibility of illness. Paranoid symptoms are indicative of an ability to change; therefore, they result in more transient violence and are negatively related to persistent violence. The symptoms were most prominent in the transient-violence group during the first week of stay; they improved rapidly and the patients were therefore less likely to continue to be violent. In contrast, neurological impairment, the organic or process component, results in a chronic, repetitive pattern of violence, an association consistent with the above-mentioned literature (15–18).

Given the special nature of the secure unit, the length of stay was an important outcome measure. The decision to transfer a patient back to his home ward was reached by the staff through clinical judgment without any methodical evaluation, but it proved to be related to measures of impairment systematically and independently assessed. Length of stay was mostly affected by factor 1, which consisted of various psychiatric symptoms and behavioral abnormalities. This finding is consistent with reports in the literature that clinicians perceive more disordered patients as being more dangerous; thus it is reported that "the more severely disordered a patient is on any mental disorder dimension . . . the higher is the overall dangerousness of the patient as perceived by the clinicians" (33).

In our study, length of stay was not related to the frequency of violence over a fixed period; it would appear that if patients show sufficient overall improvement in psychiatric symptoms and ward behaviors, they will no longer be considered dangerous even if they have been repeatedly violent.

A high percentage of patients in our study had a history of substance abuse, which has often been associated with violence. Since drug screens were not performed systematically, we cannot exclude the possibility that some patients gained access to drugs or alcohol before their transfer to the special unit. On the basis of the information available, we did not find that patients with a history of substance abuse differed from the other patients in paranoid or other psychotic symptoms on admission, nor in the resolution of these symptoms over time. It is nonetheless possible that substance use before transfer contributed to the exacerbation of the illness and to the paranoid symptoms in patients who were transiently violent.

The persistence of violence, however, cannot be attributed to substance use; once on the special unit, no patients could gain access to drugs or alcohol because they were never allowed off the ward and were closely monitored there. The chronic repetitive violence evidenced by our recidivistic patients—clusters of assaults early on admission—differed from the pattern that would be expected with use of an intoxicant. Patients with a history of substance abuse did not show more recidivistic violence or neurological impairment than the other patients.

This study dealt with a special population, inpatients whose violent behavior could not be controlled on their home wards and who were transferred to a secure care unit that provided strong deterrence for such behavior. As such, some important distinctions must be drawn between them and violent populations in other settings. These distinctions are especially important with regard to persistent violence, which in this study represents a chronic repetitive pattern and is quite different from clusters of assaults by intoxicated or acutely psychotic patients early in their hospital stay. With regard to the etiology of violence, substance abuse or general impairment and psychopathology (factor 1) probably plays a more important role for patients in the community than it did for these inpatients on the special unit.

This study underscores the need for differential treatment of violent behavior in psychiatric inpatients, as different psychopathological processes might be involved. Transient violence occurs in the context of prominent paranoid delusions and is probably a symptom of acute decompensation, while chronic, repetitive patterns of violence are associated with neurological impairment. Treatment of the underlying psychiatric disorder with antipsychotic medication may well be the primary choice for transient violence, but other pharmacological agents should be considered for recidivistic violence. ♦

Acknowledgments

This study was supported in part by grant MH-45454-03 from the National Institute of Mental Health.

References

1. Monahan J: Mental disorder and violent behavior: perceptions and evidence. American Psychologist 47:511–521, 1992
2. Volkow ND, Tancredi L: Neural substrates of violent behaviour: a preliminary study with positron emission tomography. British Journal of Psychiatry 151:668–673, 1987
3. Spellacy F: Neuropsychological differences between violent and nonviolent men. Journal of Clinical Psychology 34:49–52, 1978
4. Tardiff K, Sweillam A: Assault, suicide, and mental illness. Archives of General Psychiatry 37:164–169, 1980
5. Planansky K, Johnston R: Homicidal aggression in schizophrenic men. Acta Psychiatrica Scandinavica 55:65–73, 1977
6. Overall JE, Gorham DR: The Brief Psychiatric Rating Scale. Psychological Reports 10:799–812, 1962
7. Yesavage JA: Bipolar illness: correlates of dangerous inpatient behavior. British Journal of Psychiatry 143:554–557, 1983
8. Yesavage JA: Inpatient violence and the schizophrenic patient. Acta Psychiatrica Scandinavica 67:353–357, 1983
9. Yesavage JA, Werner PD, Becker JM, et al: Inpatient evaluation of aggression in psychiatric patients. Journal of Nervous and Mental Disease 169:299–301, 1981
10. Link BG, Cullen FT, Andrews H: The violent and illegal behavior of mental patients reconsidered. American Sociological Review 57:275–292, 1992
11. Tucker GJ, Campion EW, Kelleher PA, et al: The relationship of subtle neurologic impairments to disturbances of thinking. Psychotherapy and Psychosomatics 24:165–169, 1974
12. Tucker GJ, Campion EW, Silberfarb PM: Sensorimotor functions and cognitive disturbance in psychiatric patients. American Journal of Psychiatry 132:17–21, 1975
13. Tardiff K, Sweillam A: Assaultive behavior among chronic inpatients. American Journal of Psychiatry 139:212–215, 1982
14. Krakowski M, Volavka J, Brizer D: Psychopathology and violence: a review of literature. Comprehensive Psychiatry 27:131–148, 1986
15. Wolfgang ME: Delinquency and violence from the viewpoint of criminology, in Neural Bases of Violence and Aggression. Edited by Field W, Sweet W. St Louis, Green, 1975
16. Monroe RR, Hulfish B, Balis G, et al: Neurologic findings in recidivist aggressors, in Psychopathology and Brain Dysfunction.

Edited by Shagess C, Gershon S, Friedhoff AJ. New York, Raven, 1977

17. Lewis DO: Delinquency, psychomotor epileptic symptoms, and paranoid ideation: a triad. American Journal of Psychiatry 133:1395–1398, 1976

18. Yeudall LT: Neuropsychological concomitants of persistent criminal behavior. Research Bulletin no 29, Alberta Hospital, Edmonton, Alberta, 1979

19. Krakowski M, Convit A, Jaeger J, et al: Inpatient violence: trait and state. Journal of Psychiatric Research 23:57–64, 1989

20. Volovka J, Krakowski M: Schizophrenia and violence. Psychological Medicine 19:559–562, 1989

21. Eaton LF, Menolascino FJ: Psychiatric disorders in the mentally retarded: types, problems, and challenges. American Journal of Psychiatry 139:1297–1303, 1982

22. Menolascino FJ, Ruedrich S, Golden C, et al: Schizophrenia in the mentally retarded. Psychiatric Hospital 12:16, 21–25, 1985

23. Convit A, Jaeger J, Lin S, et al: Prediction of violence in psychiatric inpatients, in Biological Contributions to Crime Causation. Edited by Moffit TE, Mednick SA. Amsterdam, Martinus Nijhoff, 1988

24. Kay S: Social Participation Rating Scale. Psychological Documents 14:27, 1984

25. Guy W: ECDEU Assessment Manual for Psychopharmacology. Rockville, Md, Department of Health and Human Services, 1976

26. Crow TJ: Two syndromes of schizophrenia? Trends in the Neurosciences 5:351–354, 1982

27. Garmezy N: Process and reactive schizophrenia: some conceptions and issues. Schizophrenia Bulletin 2:30–74, 1970

28. Crow TJ: Positive and negative schizophrenia symptoms and the role of dopamine. British Journal of Psychiatry 139:251–253, 1981

29. Quitkin F, Rifkin A, Klein DF: Neurologic soft signs in schizophrenia and character disorder. Archives of General Psychiatry 33:845–853, 1976

30. Kay S: Significance of the positive-negative distinction in schizophrenia. Schizophrenia Bulletin 16:635–652, 1990

31. Strauss M, Sirotkin R, Grisel J: Length of hospitalization and rate of readmission of paranoid and nonparanoid schizophrenics. Journal of Consulting and Clinical Psychology 42:105–110, 1974

32. Tsuang M, Winokur G: Criteria for subtyping schizophrenia: clinical differentiation of hebephrenic and paranoid schizophrenia. Archives of General Psychiatry 31:43–47, 1974

33. Segal SP, Watson MA, Goldfinger SM, et al: Civil commitment in the psychiatric emergency room, II: mental disorder indicators and three dangerousness criteria. Archives of General Psychiatry 45:753–758, 1988

Involuntary Community Treatment of People Who Are Violent and Mentally Ill: A Legal Analysis

Christopher Slobogin, J.D., LL.M.

In the last three decades virtually every state has adopted statutory language requiring that involuntary psychiatric treatment take place in the least restrictive setting, or the least restrictive "available" setting. This requirement derives from the constitutional doctrine, developed in the mid-20th century in First Amendment cases (1), that government intervention should generally be limited to the minimum necessary to achieve the government's aim. This paper describes the three major legal mechanisms associated with this doctrine as they apply to people who are violent and mentally ill, examines the constitutionality of these mechanisms, and discusses the extent to which the right to refuse treatment and various procedural rights should be recognized within this framework.

Three major legal mechanisms exist for providing involuntary community treatment to people who are violent and mentally disabled: outpatient commitment, preventive commitment, and conditional release from a hospital. In most states, predicted deterioration is either the explicit or the de facto criterion for involuntary community treatment. However, the constitutionality of this standard has been the subject of considerable debate, centering on whether involuntary treatment in the community requires a showing of imminent dangerousness and an overt act of dangerousness and whether a person who is not dangerous solely because of treatment may be committed. The author suggests that the predicted deterioration standard is constitutional, but only if it is accompanied by limitations on the duration of commitment and proof that involuntary treatment is necessary to prevent danger to self or others. The author also discusses whether a person committed under the predicted deterioration standard has the right to refuse treatment and whether persons hospitalized after being committed to involuntary community treatment should receive a hearing.

When this paper was published **Mr. Slobogin** *was professor of law at the University of Florida College of Law in Gainesville. From the July 1994 issue of* Hospital and Community Psychiatry *(volume 45, pages 685–689).*

Legal mechanisms

The most obvious way of implementing the requirement for the least restrictive alternative treatment in the commitment process is to require commitment to an outpatient program rather than to a hospital whenever possible. About half the states provide this option by statute (2). This type of commitment, called outpatient commitment in this paper, is meant to provide an alternative disposition to inpatient treatment for individuals who meet the traditional commitment criteria of dangerousness to self or others.

Community treatment of people who are violent and mentally ill may also be provided through two other mechanisms—preventive commitment and conditional release. Although they too appear to implement the objective of providing treatment in the least restrictive alternative, these interventions actually derive from other agendas.

Preventive commitment is a relatively new innovation that exists in only a few states. In contrast to outpatient commitment, preventive commitment permits commitment to outpatient treatment (and in some states, to inpatient treatment as well) of persons who do not yet meet the usual commitment criteria, but will soon do so if intervention does not take place.

The criterion for commitment under preventive commitment statutes might be called a "predicted deterioration" standard. For instance, Hawaii allows outpatient commitment for an individual who "has been imminently dangerous to self or others as a result of a severe mental disorder" and is now in need of treatment "to prevent a relapse or deterioration which would predictably result" in the individual's becoming "imminently dangerous" (3,4). Apparently, preventive commitment statutes were enacted because of concerns about the growing number of homeless people with mental disorders who could not be hospitalized under strict commitment criteria, concerns among psychiatrists and mental health professionals about over-legalization of the mental health system, and advocacy by parents' groups, particularly the National Alliance for the Mentally Ill, which have allied with mental health professionals to press for less strict commitment standards (5).

The third type of involuntary community treatment, which is usually called conditional release, has been available for some time in about 40 states (6). It involves continued supervision of a person who has been released from the hospital. Under this type of community program, the hospital or, in criminal cases, the court, informs the conditionally released person of the release conditions (for example, reporting to a clinic for medication). Violation of one or more of these conditions will usually trigger rehospitalization, either summarily or after a hearing. In contrast to outpatient commitment, which is designed as an alternative to inpatient commitment, and preventive commitment, which is anticipatory, conditional release is primarily intended to test the treated individual's ability to function in the community under supervision and to free up hospital beds.

The three mechanisms for treating mentally ill people in the community thus stem from different policy goals. However, on close inspection, they are similar in both their substantive and their procedural features. In terms of substantive criteria, a person supposedly is not eligible for outpatient commitment unless he or she meets the usual criteria for commitment to inpatient treatment, whereas preventive commitment and conditional release can be triggered by something less. However, because a person who is currently or imminently dangerous to self or others usually cannot be treated on an outpatient basis, the only type of "violent" person who is actually eligible for the first type of commitment is one who will eventually (rather than immediately) harm others. Presumably, this is the same type of "violent" person affected by preventive commitment and conditional release provisions.

In terms of procedural features, differences between the three mechanisms are more likely to occur. In particular, conditional release is less likely to be triggered by a judicial hearing than either outpatient commitment or preventive commitment. But in most respects the majority of states do not differentiate between the mechanisms procedurally (7). The few differences that do exist will be highlighted in later discussion.

The predicted deterioration standard

Each of the three mechanisms for treating people on an outpatient basis permits involuntary treatment of individuals who are not currently dangerous but rather may soon be—preventive commitment and conditional release explicitly, and outpatient commitment implicitly. The primary issue addressed here is whether involuntary treatment based on this predicted deterioration standard is justified as a constitutional or policy matter. The courts have addressed three issues that might affect the constitutionality of the standard: the imminence requirement, the overt act requirement, and the so-called "synthetic sanity" issue.

Several courts have held that due process requires a finding of imminent dangerousness for civil commitment to occur (8–10). For instance, in the leading case of *Lessard v. Schmidt* (8), a three-judge federal district court held that involuntary commitment is constitutionally justified only if there is an "extreme likelihood that if the person is not confined he will do immediate harm to himself or others." This holding would presumably eliminate the possibility of a predicted deterioration standard, since the danger that the latter standard contemplates is relatively remote. The courts that have required a showing of imminence seem to do so on two grounds: the Millsian proposition that, absent a clear and present danger, the state cannot engage in the "massive deprivation of liberty" associated with commitment and the assumption that forecasts of long-term danger are less reliable than short-term predictions. Other courts, however, have rejected an imminence requirement (11–13), preferring merely proof of "a substantial risk of dangerous conduct within the reasonably foreseeable future" (12).

To assist in the prediction of dangerousness and perhaps also to avoid the possibility of punishment for the status of being mentally ill and dangerous, *Lessard* also held that proof of a recent overt act evidencing dangerousness is necessary for involuntary treatment. If a significant overt act must be proven, a "predicted deterioration" standard, which merely requires proof that such an act may occur, might be difficult to sustain. Many other lower courts have followed the precedent set by *Lessard* (14,15), including some that have rejected the imminence requirement (13). Others, however, have merely endorsed the dangerousness criterion, without requiring either proof of imminence or proof of an overt act (16–18). It is also worth noting that a majority of state statutes do not require proof of an overt act for involuntary commitment (19).

The litigation most directly related to the viability of the predicted deterioration standard deals with the legality of committing people who are thought to be nondangerous solely because of treatment (usually medication) they are receiving. The mental condition of such people is sometimes called "synthetic sanity," although the term is probably inappropriate from the clinical perspective (20). Most courts go so far as to permit institutionalization under such circumstances (21,22). Others do not permit inpatient care in synthetic sanity cases but still allow the state to subject the individual to "probationary conditions" on an outpatient basis, as contemplated under the conditional release programs described above (23,24).

Considering the various positions staked out above, the constitutionality of the predicted deterioration standard is unclear. Courts that insist on the imminence and overt act requirements would presumably be hostile to the standard, while courts that reject those requirements and permit commitment in synthetic sanity cases might accept it. The normative question is whether the liberty interest of a person who is said to meet the predicted deterioration standard outweighs the state's interests in preventing whatever harm may be caused by that person if intervention does not take place. Although the individual clearly has an interest in avoiding unnecessary coercive treatment, the state also has a valid interest in ensuring that an individual who otherwise will be violent is treated appropriately. Probably the most supportable position on this issue is that the predicted deterioration standard is constitutional, but only if it is carefully limited. The following discussion fleshes out this compromise position from the perspective of the imminence requirement, the overt act requirement, and the synthetic sanity dilemma.

A compromise position

As Brooks (25) has argued, dangerousness is best conceptualized as a multifactor construct, involving the nature of the anticipated harm, its probability of occurrence, the frequency with which it may occur, and its imminence. Under this formulation, the imminence of the harm is only one of many factors considered in deciding whether a mentally ill person should be subject to involuntary state intervention for treatment. Thus, for instance, if the harm likely to be caused by the person is significant and probable or is likely to occur frequently, it probably does not need to be imminent to justify the person's commitment.

The considerations underlying the imminence requirement should still be influential, however, in determining the length of commitment. The predicted deterioration standard could easily create a class of patients who never escape the state's control because their dangerousness is always just around the corner (26,27). If we allow commitment under such a standard, we should also require that persons who are so committed be eligible for automatic release from outpatient commitment after a certain time period, unless their dangerousness becomes imminent while they are committed (28).

The overt act requirement can be subjected to similar analysis. The argument that such a requirement is necessary to avoid confinement on the basis of a person's status does not work; even commitment on proof of an overt act is confinement due to status—the status of being mentally ill and the status of being dangerous. As for the argument that the requirement is needed to ensure reliable predictions, recent theoretical work on dangerousness suggests the contrary (29, but see 30).

In any event, a petition for outpatient or preventive commitment is almost always precipitated by overt behavior. The real issue in these two contexts is not whether an overt act is required but what type of "acts" justify a prediction of dangerousness. Does the act have to be one of physical violence, or may it be verbal only? Does it have to communicate a violent intent, or may it merely show evidence of a pattern of behavior that has led to violent behavior in the past? These latter questions are ultimately empirical ones, and no attempt to answer them will be made here.

The analysis of the overt act requirement changes somewhat for conditional release, because in this context the person's nonviolence triggers eligibility for the mechanism. Continued state control via conditional release is sought not because of recent violence but because, without involuntary treatment, the person is likely to revert to the patterns that led to the original commitment weeks, months, or even years earlier. The "synthetic sanity" cases posit that the state interest in continued control of such individuals supersedes the individual's interest in being free of this control. Although this stance is questionable when the intervention is institutionalization, it is more justifiable when the state seeks outpatient treatment, in which the infringement on liberty interests is usually not as significant.

Nonetheless, to justify conditional, as opposed to outright, release, the state should have to show that the person's history demonstrates a failure to conform to the specified treatment regimen when left unsupervised and that the absence of treatment results in violent behavior. And, as with outpatient and preventive commitment, conditional release should probably have defined time limits.

In short, the ideas underlying the imminent dangerousness and overt act requirements, although not directly applicable to involuntary community treatment, can be reshaped to place proof and duration limitations on outpatient, preventive, and conditional commitment. Even with these limitations, however, the predicted deterioration standard faces one final challenge: does it effectively implement the state's objective, that is, reducing the risk of violence? If violence is just as likely with the standard as without it, it cannot be countenanced as a justification for coercively treating competent mentally ill people thought to be dangerous. To explore this issue, one must examine, at a minimum, two other issues: whether persons subjected to involuntary outpatient treatment can refuse the treatment and, assuming they cannot, the methods the state can use to enforce its treatment plan.

Right to refuse treatment

In *Washington v. Harper* (31), the Supreme Court upheld a state prison policy that permitted involuntary medication of prisoners who suffered from a "mental disorder" and who are "gravely disabled" or pose a "likelihood of serious harm" to themselves, others, or property. No finding of incompetency to make a treatment decision was required by the policy.

In light of *Harper*, the states can probably impose psychoactive medication as a condition of outpatient treatment for persons who are mentally ill and evidence a "likelihood of serious harm," even if they are competent to make treatment decisions. Against this extension of *Harper*, one might argue that a convicted person's interest in avoiding medication is weaker than that of a person committed to involuntary treatment in the community, while the state's interest in medicating prisoners is stronger than its interest in medicating a person so committed. But a court's most likely conclusion would be, to the contrary, that a committed person has no stronger interest in avoiding medication than a prisoner and that the state's interest in forcibly medicating dangerous individuals who will be at large in the community is even stronger than its interest in medicating those who are in prison.

Even if one accepts the latter argument, however, the *Harper* decision does not mean that a person committed under a predicted deterioration standard has no right to refuse treatment. By definition, such a person is not, at least at the time of commitment, imminently violent. To the extent that this is true, an absolute right to refuse may exist for the competent patient, thus undercutting the preventive rationale for the standard.

To address this anomaly, courts might construe the phrase "likelihood of serious harm" in *Harper* to encompass harm that results from deterioration. But even this move would not entirely eliminate the right to refuse medication for potentially violent individuals. *Harper* made clear that the treatment imposed over a prisoner's objection must be in the inmate's "medical interest."

In *Riggins v. Nevada* (32), decided two years after *Harper*, the Supreme Court appeared to interpret this idea in a manner that places significant limitations on the state's authority to treat involuntarily. *Riggins* held that the state may not overmedicate an individual during his capital murder trial. In the course of justifying its decision, the court stated: "Nevada certainly would have satisfied due process if the prosecution had demonstrated and the District Court had found that treatment with antipsychotic medications was medically appropriate and, considering less intrusive alternatives, essential for the sake of Riggins' own safety or the safety of others. Similarly, the State might have been able to justify medically appropriate, involuntary treatment with the drug by establishing that it could not obtain an adjudication of Riggins' guilt or innocence by using less intrusive means."

Although this language seems to affirm the *Harper* holding that the state may forcibly medicate an individual if necessary to curb violence, it also suggests that, if other less intrusive means of accomplishing this goal are available, the individual may require the state to use them.

Ensuring compliance

Several different judicial and administrative models for ensuring that individuals comply with outpatient treatment and medication plans have been envisioned (34–38). Evaluating their relative worth as means of achieving the state's aim of reducing violence is beyond the scope of this paper. However, this paper will address one issue that should be common to all of them: the proper procedure for revoking or terminating outpatient treatment and recommitting or committing the individual to an inpatient facility. Courts that have analyzed this issue have focused on the analogy to revocation of parole. The leading decision is *Morrissey v. Brewer* (39), in which the Supreme Court held that the "conditional liberty" of paroled criminals entitles them to preliminary and final revocation hearings, the right to advance notice of the proceedings, the right to confront accusers, and, in "complex" revocation proceedings, the right to counsel as well.

Some courts, contrasting the therapeutic rationale of hospitalization with the punitive intent behind parole revocation, have held that *Morrissey* does not apply to outpatient treatment, at least to revocation of conditional release. These courts have thus upheld automatic rehospitalization of the outpatient who has violated a condition of treatment, although they also note that the person can always subsequently challenge a detention through a writ of habeas corpus (40,41). Other courts have permitted emergency detention but then required a prompt *Morrissey*-type hearing to determine whether hospitalization was warranted (7,42–45).

Comparing revocation of parole with revocation of conditional release (or with hospitalization after an initial outpatient commitment) is problematic. In many cases, hospitalization will be less punitive and of shorter duration than imprisonment after revocation of parole. At the same time, the state has clear authority to incarcerate the paroled criminal defendant for the time period denominated by the sentence, regardless of whether an additional antisocial act has been committed. In contrast, the state does not have authority to confine the unconvicted mentally ill person unless he or she is dangerous to self or others. Thus an erroneous determination in the latter situation is more consequential. At the least, persons on outpatient status who are subsequently hospitalized should receive a hearing within a short time after detention.

Conclusions

A concise statement of the law regarding outpatient treatment of potentially violent mentally ill individuals is impossible because the law is unclear. However, several major themes explored in this paper can be summarized.

First, community treatment of potentially violent mentally ill persons is likely to employ one of three mechanisms: outpatient commitment (commitment to an outpatient program under the criteria for commitment to inpatient treatment), preventive commitment (outpatient commitment under a predicted deterioration standard), and conditional release from a hospital (outpatient commitment based on continued satisfaction of certain conditions).

Second, whether these forms of commitment are constitutional is not clear. At the least, they should be permitted only on clear and convincing proof that the person being committed is mentally ill and is likely to cause serious harm to others unless subjected to a specified treatment regimen. Such proof should require evidence that violent actions will occur if the person is not treated. If commitment occurs, the treatment should be specifically limited in time, unless subsequent behavior suggests that the person is imminently dangerous.

Third, a competent person subject to commitment under the above criterion may have an "absolute" right to refuse psychoactive medication; alternatively, such a right exists when the medication is not the least intrusive effective means of preventing or reducing the person's potential for violence. Similarly, the involuntary aspects of the treatment regimen should relate solely to the diminution of the patient's potential for violence.

Fourth, emergency detention of an outpatient who has violated a treatment condition is probably permissible. However, due process probably requires a prompt postdetention hearing that meets, at the least, the requirements established by *Morrissey v. Brewer,* including the right to advance notice of the proceedings, the right to counsel in complex cases, and the right to confront accusers. ◆

References

1. Shelton v Tucker, 364 US 479 (1960)
2. Keilitz I, Conn D, Giampetro A: Least restrictive treatment of involuntary patients: translating concepts into practice. St Louis University Law Review 29:691–745, 1985
3. Hawaii Revised Statutes, sec 334–121 (1985)
4. General Statutes of North Carolina, sec 122C–271 (a) (1) (1989)
5. Stefan SB: Preventive commitment: the concept and its pitfalls. Mental Disability Law Reporter 11:288–290, 1987
6. Brakel S, Parry J, Weiner B: The Mentally Disabled and the Law. Chicago, American Bar Foundation, 1985
7. Hinds JT: Involuntary outpatient commitment for the chronically mentally ill. Nebraska Law Review 69:346–412, 1990
8. Lessard v Schmidt, 349 F Supp 1078 (ED Wis 1972)
9. Suzuki v Alba, 438 F Supp 1006 (D Hawaii 1977)
10. Mignone v Vincent, 411 F Supp 1386, 1389 (SD NY 1976)
11. Hatcher v Wachtel, 269 SE 2d 849,852 (W Va 1980)
12. Commonwealth v Nassar, 380 Mass 908, 406 NE 2d 1286 (1980)
13. In re Harris, 98 Wash 2d 276, 654 P 2d 109,113 (1982)
14. Lynch v Baxley, 386 F Supp 378 (MD Ala 1974)
15. Commonwealth ex rel Finken v Roop, 234 Pa Super 155,339 A 2d 764 (1975)
16. United States ex rel Matthew v Nelson, No 72-C-2194 (ND Ill Aug 18, 1975), noted in Loyola University of Chicago Law Journal 7:507, 1976
17. People v Sansone, 18 Ill App 3d 315,317, 309 NE 2d 733,735 (1974)
18. In re Salem, 228 SE 2d 649 (NC Ct App 1976)
19. Reisner R, Slobogin C: Law and the Mental Health System: Criminal and Civil Aspects. St Paul, Minn, West, 1990
20. Gutheil TG, Appelbaum PS: "Mind control," "synthetic sanity," "artificial competence," and genuine confusion: legally relevant actions of antipsychotic medications. Hofstra Law Review 12:77–120, 1983
21. Wolonsky v Balson, 58 Ohio App 2d 25, 387 NE 2d 625 (1976)
22. People v De Anda, 114 Cal App 3d 488, 170 Cal Rptr 830, 833–837 (1980)
23. State v Collins, 381 So 2d 449 (La 1980)
24. Criminal Justice Mental Health Standard 7-7.4(d). Washington, DC, American Bar Association, 1989
25. Brooks A: Psychiatry and Mental Health Systems. Boston, Little Brown, 1974
26. McNiel DE, Binder RL: Judgments of dangerousness in emergency civil commitment. American Journal of Psychiatry 144:197–200, 1987
27. Durham ML, LaFond JQ: The empirical consequences and policy implications of broadening the statutory criteria for civil commitment. Yale Law and Policy Review 3:395–446, 1985
28. Stromberg CD, Stone AA: A model state law on civil commitment of the mentally ill. Harvard Journal on Legislation 20:275–396, 1983
29. Litwack TR, Schlesinger LB: Assessing and predicting violence: research, law, and applications, in Handbook of Forensic Psychology. Edited by Weiner IB, Hess AK. New York, Wiley, 1987
30. Monahan J: The Clinical Prediction of Violent Behavior. Washington, DC, National Institute of Mental Health, 1980
31. Washington v Harper, 110 S Ct 1028 (1990)
32. Riggins v Nevada, 112 S Ct 1810 (1992)
33. Dvoskin J, Steadman H: Using intensive case management to reduce violence by mentally ill persons in the community. Hospital and Community Psychiatry 45:679–684, 1994
34. Wexler DB: Health care compliance principles and the insanity acquittee conditional release process. Criminal Law Bulletin 27:18–41, 1991
35. Meichenbaum D, Turk DC: Facilitating Treatment Adherence: A Practitioner's Guidebook. New York, Plenum, 1987
36. Oregon Revised Statutes, secs 161.327 to 161.336 (1981)
37. Rogers JL, Bloom JD, Mason SM: After Oregon's insanity defense: a comparison of conditional release and hospitalization. International Journal of Law and Psychiatry 5:391–403, 1982
38. Lamb HR, Weinberger LE, Gross BH: Court-mandated outpatient treatment for insanity acquittees: clinical philosophy and implementation. Hospital and Community Psychiatry 39:1080–1084, 1988
39. Morrissey v Brewer, 408 US 471 (1972)
40. Dietrich v Brooks, 27 Or App 821, 558 P 2d 357 (1976)
41. In re Richardson, 481 A 2d 473 (DC 1984)
42. GT v Vermont, Ver S Ct, no 92-941 (1992)
43. Application of True v Department of Health and Welfare, 103 Idaho 151, 645 P 2d 891 (1982)
44. In re Peterson, 360 NW 2d 33 (Minn 1984)
45. Birls v Wallis, 619 F Supp 481 (MD Ala 1985)

Using Intensive Case Management to Reduce Violence by Mentally Ill Persons in the Community

Joel A. Dvoskin, Ph.D.
Henry J. Steadman, Ph.D.

Aggressive and intensive case management and a comprehensive array of community support services are the keys to reducing the risk of violence by people with serious mental illness in the community. The authors describe the elements of intensive case management for potentially violent clients, including use of individual case managers responsible for small caseloads, 24-hour availability of case managers, and strong linkages to agencies providing mental health services, substance abuse treatment, and social services as well as to the criminal justice system. They summarize the results of three recent studies of intensive case management programs suggesting that this intervention is effective in reducing clients' dangerousness in the community. They discuss cultural and human resource issues that affect planning of intensive case management services. Intensive case managers need to be "boundary spanners" with the training, experience, and personality to bridge the often-broad gap between human service and criminal justice systems.

On December 13, 1992, nearly one-third of the television program *60 Minutes* was devoted to the case of Larry Hogue, a 48-year-old African-American man living in New York City. According to the press (1,3), he annually received $36,000 in disability payments from the Department of Veterans Affairs, but he did not use the benefits to gain housing or other basic necessities. Instead, he spent his income on alcohol, marijuana, and crack cocaine, and he was chronically homeless.

It was reported that when he was under the influence of these substances, his behavior terrorized the entire Upper West Side of Manhattan. He was reported to throw garbage and feces at passers-by, destroy property, and light fires under automobiles or stuff rags in their gas tanks. He was once convicted in a jury trial of reckless endangerment for pushing a young girl in front of an oncoming truck, which barely managed to stop without hitting her. Yet, when he was civilly committed to inpatient psychiatric treatment and was away from street drugs, it was reported that his behavior became peaceful and even docile, and hospital administrators concluded that he should be released.

If there are treatments available that will reduce violence associated with mental disorder, how can they be delivered most effectively? How can the Larry Hogues across the U.S. be managed while both their rights to liberty, due process, and least restrictive setting and the public's right to be safe are properly balanced? This paper examines these questions and proposes that intensive case management is an effective intervention to reduce the risk of violent behavior by mentally ill persons in the community. Case management can be an appropriate strategy for risk management if individual case managers are responsible for small caseloads and if a comprehensive array of services are available in the community.

Case managers as risk managers

Many mental health systems in the U.S. are not able to offer truly comprehensive services and thus have difficulty providing the continuous

---

When this paper was published **Dr. Dvoskin** *was associate commissioner for forensic services with the New York State Office of Mental Health in Albany.* **Dr. Steadman** *was president of Policy Research Associates in Delmar, New York. From the July 1994 issue of Hospital and Community Psychiatry (volume 45, pages 679–684).*

care that is needed by mentally ill people in the community, including those who sometimes engage in violent behavior. However, effective intensive case management that coordinates the services of a wide variety of community agencies can facilitate their living safely in the community. The case manager, with appropriate caseloads, works to manage both the risks faced by the client and the risk the client could possibly pose to the community. The organizing theme of all case management services is the management of a wide variety of risks. We concentrate here on only one of those risks, the risk of violence associated with mental illness in the community.

People with mental illness, especially those with histories of violent behavior, most often require continuous rather than episodic care. The medical paradigm that treatment is provided only when symptoms are evident is inconsistent with effective community supervision and support of persons with mental illness who have a history of violent behavior. Such persons need regular monitoring, especially when symptoms are absent or at a low ebb, to contain the individual and situational factors that may result in violence.

One of the most important roles of the case manager as risk manager is teaching clients to recognize and respond to high-risk situations, the nature of which varies from client to client. Case managers can help clients to gain insight into the kinds of situations that have led to violence in the past and to develop strategies for avoiding such situations and ways of resolving them if they cannot be avoided.

Definitions of case management abound and include many different processes and responsibilities (4–6). However, all models of case management involve the case manager as "a vehicle for implementing continuity in the care of mentally ill persons" (4). Our purpose here is not to assess the value of various models, which has been addressed in a useful review by Solomon (5). Rather, we will discuss case management as it relates to issues of violence, as both a service modality and an operating system that seeks to organize and synthesize elements of the mental health, social services, and criminal justice systems.

> *Case managers can help clients to gain insight into the kinds of situations that have led to violence in the past and to develop strategies for avoiding such situations and ways of resolving them if they cannot be avoided.*

During the last 15 years, case management has evolved as a service modality that usually targets persons with serious mental illness who have been ill served by or unwilling to participate in the generic mental health system. In New York State, for example, the State Office of Mental Health recently began a major intensive case management program for persons with mental illness who are frequent users of expensive psychiatric services such as emergency rooms and inpatient care.

Surles and colleagues (7) have identified eight characteristics of this initiative. First, the client (as opposed to a particular treatment program) is the central focus for the case manager. Second, persons are "nominated" locally for participation in the program by those responsible for treatment. Third, persons cannot be removed from the program roster for "failure to improve." Fourth, caseloads are limited to ten persons per case manager. Fifth, activities are expected to occur in the client's community. Sixth, case managers are expected to be accessible. Seventh, case managers serve as advocates and develop support for clients, who are encouraged to express their own goals and concerns. Eighth, services are not time limited.

So far we have been discussing case management as a system of services. However, there is debate in the field about the optimum way of delivering services. In this paper, the primary mode of service delivery we describe relies on each client's being assigned an individual case manager. Stein (8) recently proposed an alternative service delivery model involving continuous care teams interdisciplinary teams with low patient-to-staff ratios that operate seven days a week. Stein recommended that these teams should not be thought of as treatment, rehabilitation, or case management teams but as vehicles for providing whatever service or practical assistance a patient requires. He suggested that because the continuous care team provides most services itself and brokers for only a few, services are integrated and responsive to the client's current needs.

We suggest that continuous care teams, as proposed by Stein, constitute a comprehensive outpatient treatment program. Although we agree with Stein that a full array of integrated and responsive services could remove the need for an individual case manager, such ideal systems exists in few places in the United States. In the absence of such systems, we remain convinced of the necessity for individual case managers who integrate services through creative brokering and advocacy. Whether some version of the proposed continuous care team is ultimately preferable awaits future research. In the meantime, intensive case management programs that rely on individual case managers constitute the most practical method of managing violence associated with mental illness in the community.

Specific clients must be identified and assigned by name to individual case managers. Such assignments are perhaps the most important facet of case management and its greatest value because they prevent case managers from disavowing responsibility for clients who may engage in violent, criminal, psychotic, embarrassing, or threatening behavior. Although case managers may occasionally need to rely on the resources of the criminal justice system or on emergency psychiatric services to respond to clients in potentially violent situations, they continue to be responsible for providing the person with case management and support services, even if the person goes to jail.

Many persons with mental illness who frequently interact with the criminal justice system have been disenfranchised for a variety of reasons. Many are from lower social classes, either because their family of origin was poor or because their mental illness has forestalled employment necessary to maintain social status. Many are unmarried, young, and homeless and may view the mental health and social services systems as their enemy.

Obviously, engaging such a group in treatment is difficult. Mental health systems have traditionally attempted to do so by developing a finite variety of treatment modalities and attempting to fit clients into those services. Such an approach may be suitable for clients who are passive, dependent, and compliant. However, persons with mental illness who have recently come into contact with the criminal justice system because they have been violent are likely to be active, independent, and unwilling to obey orders. Furthermore, many of these people have not had the long hospital stays that characterized an earlier generation of people with serious mental illness. Patients with long hospital stays often learned compliant behaviors that prepared them to accept traditional community mental health services. People with mental illness who are at risk for violent behavior not only may lack these compliant behaviors but may actively antagonize providers in community mental health programs (9).

As in New York's intensive case management program, case managers in effective programs for potentially violent clients must have extremely low caseloads and must be available to clients 24 hours a day, either individually or via teams. Many violent acts and arrests occur in the evening or during the night, when traditional programs are closed. The case management program must have the ability to respond quickly when violence is part of a psychiatric crisis that occurs during these off hours.

One important reason for having low caseloads for intensive case managers is that developing a personal relationship with a client takes a great deal of time and individualized attention. Furthermore, most of this work does not take place in offices, but on the streets and other locations where the clients live and hang out. The importance of this relationship cannot be overstated. One of the simple ways violence can be avoided is to talk about anger. For someone who is socially isolated or whose entire peer support group is made up of people who repetitively act out violent thoughts and feelings, this modulating and inhibiting does not exist. Often, the ability simply to express anger verbally to someone who is perceived as being interested can allow a person an alternative to violent behavior that may not otherwise exist.

Another advantage of a personal relationship with a case manager is that it offers clients an appropriate way to seek more intense treatment services. Tragically, some clients who feel they need to be hospitalized may believe that the only way to receive such help is to commit a violent act. Clients who can go to their case manager for help may no longer feel the need to be violent.

Sometimes, of course, a poor personal match between an individual client and a case manager may occur. Case managers should meet as teams to flexibly address the needs of clients who might be better off with a case manager from a different gender, race, culture, or generation.

Before accepting case management and other services, clients first ask themselves "What's in it for me?" Clients who perceive the case manager as an agent of the state whose sole intention is to make the client "toe the line" will be unlikely to invest any effort in forming a relationship with a case manager. The case manager must thus be seen as an advocate for the client even if other agencies such as the criminal justice system are at the same time dealing with the client in more coercive or authoritarian ways.

What form should this advocacy take? Certainly, case managers should not suggest to clients that they need not be held accountable for criminal or violent acts. However, other forms of advocacy are both necessary and appropriate. For example, as Massaro (10) and others have pointed out, health care for people with serious mental illness is often quite deficient. Case managers could advocate for clients in this area by helping them apply for Medicaid and gain access to a physician or other health care professional. The case manager could assist the client in obtaining other human services and entitlements, such as Social Security Disability Insurance, Supplemental Security Income, or food stamps, and in enrolling in and seeking resources to fund training in their desired vocation.

Case managers may have additional options, depending on the particular provisions of the case management program in which they work. For example, New York's intensive case management program provides service dollars that are intended to be used to meet a range of clients' needs, not only those related to traditional clinical concerns. A case manager may help a client use this money to make a rent payment and thus make a tenuous housing situation more permanent.

Linkages to other systems

To assist severely mentally ill clients in gaining access to the services they need, a case manager must be familiar with the services offered by departments of social services, mental health agencies, medical or health providers, and criminal justice agencies. The case manager may be the client's only social and constructive link to these systems, which have very different goals and practices and use very different terms. Case managers must be able to facilitate communication and cooperation among these agencies. The case manager must have the authority to convene meetings of appropriate staff from each service agency when necessary. Agencies' support for such meetings can be confirmed through interagency agreements or memoranda of understanding.

For clients who are at high risk of becoming violent, convenient access to services is especially important.

For a client who is known to respond to homelessness with violent or criminal behavior, being put on a two-year waiting list for subsidized housing is of little help. Although one may debate the moral propriety of giving someone high-priority access to services simply because of violent or criminal behavior, some spots in community support programs should be reserved for clients who present the highest risk to both their own and the community's safety. Such alternatives are especially necessary for clients whose behavior has not escalated to the level at which other coercive measures such as involuntary civil commitment or incarceration are legally justified.

For the client, linkages to the criminal justice system are as important as linkages to the mental health and human service delivery systems. The importance of case managers' working cooperatively with police and criminal justice agencies cannot be overstated. Case managers for high-risk clients must be able to converse fluently in the sometimes idiosyncratic language of the criminal justice system. They must be seen by police and officials in other criminal justice agencies not as helping people with mental illness avoid responsibility for crime, but rather as partners whose main vocational goal is to help make the community safer.

Case managers with links to the criminal justice system may be able to use criminal justice sanctions to facilitate potentially violent clients' adherence to treatment. Judges may release a defendant with mental illness before trial through a variety of mechanisms, including conditional probation, release on one's own recognizance, and adjudication in contemplation of dismissal, on the condition that the person is actively participating in mental health programming. Many judges have expressed to us their frustration over not being able to use these mechanisms for release more frequently because they feel there is no one to accept responsibility for organizing such programming. Judges are often as uncomfortable with the nomenclature and organization of the mental health system as mental health professionals are with that of the legal and criminal justice systems.

Probation and parole officers are important treatment allies. In addition to having the role of oversight and enforcement, parole officers provide important social supports for many of their clients. Most probation and parole officers view engaging a client in education or vocational training as important as monitoring their adherence to the conditions of their release.

However, parole and probation officers typically have caseloads that are far too large for them to adequately address the needs of mentally ill clients at high risk for violence. In addition, parole and probation officers are not likely to be able to negotiate the mental health service delivery system and are usually very grateful for the assistance of case managers. On the other hand, parole and probation officers can provide an external structure that may increase the chances that a client will adhere to an agreed-on treatment plan.

Outcome research

To date, little research has focused specifically on violence reduction as an outcome of case management. However, one study of New York State's intensive case management program (11) and two reports on forensic clients (12,13) strongly suggest that intensive case management services are effective in safely serving potentially violent clients in the community.

In an evaluation of New York's statewide intensive case management program (11), follow-up data on a variety of community functioning variables were gathered on 5,121 adult clients who received services through the program between 1989 and 1992. Some clients were followed for as long as 18 months. Results on measures of harmful behavior, antisocial behavior, and alcohol and drug abuse suggest that the program was effective in reducing clients' dangerousness in the community. Overall scores on the three measures decreased significantly for patients followed for 18 months. In addition, scores on the measures of harmful behavior and alcohol and drug abuse decreased significantly between entry and six months in the program.

The two studies of forensic populations used rearrest as a proxy measure for violent or harmful behavior. The first study assessed the effectiveness of an assertive case management program for mentally ill offenders on probation from a provincial correctional center in Vancouver, British Columbia (12). Case managers in the program each had caseloads of about ten clients, and clients received a minimum of 24 months of intensive case management. The study included a comparison group of offenders who were eligible for the program but who could not be fit into available program slots, declined to participate, or resided outside the Vancouver area. The comparison group was followed through agency records for 36 months.

During the first six months of the study, the clients who received case management averaged eight days in jail, compared with 51 days for the comparison group. At 12 months, the case management group averaged 40 days in jail, compared with 137 days for the comparison group. For the full 18 months of the study, the case management group averaged 80 jail days, while the comparison group averaged nearly three times that number (214 days). All of these differences were statistically significant, indicating the effectiveness of intensive case management in substantially reducing jail days.

A similar finding emerged from the recent evaluation of Project Action in Texas (13). From 1990 to 1992, six case managers coordinated services for 229 adult offenders released from the Harris County criminal justice system. Most of the data on the project do not relate specifically to the issues of violence. However, the evaluation showed that 75 percent of the program participants had no arrests within one year of entry into the program, 92 percent did not return to state prison, and 80 percent of the program participants who were on parole had no parole violations.

These studies are far from definitive, but they do provide preliminary empirical support for an association between intensive case management and reduced violent behavior by high-risk clients in the community.

Service planning
The case manager for a potentially violent client must be viewed as a member of any treatment team that interacts with the client. The team should assess both individual clients' strengths and their weaknesses. For example, it is quite common for a client's above-average intelligence to be viewed as an impediment to treatment. Phrases such as "too smart for his own good" and "manipulative" often appear in the records of such clients. It is ironic and unfortunate that what for most people would be deemed a strength has been considered a weakness by the mental health care providers who claim to help such clients. The presence of the case manager on the treatment team can encourage mental health care providers to enlist the client's street survival skills as important strengths that can foster rather than impede the person's recovery.

Substance abuse treatment. A full discussion of substance abuse treatment is well beyond the scope of this paper. However, in some jurisdictions, as many as 80 percent of people arrested are reported to have illegal drugs or alcohol in their systems at the time of the arrest (14). Moreover, awareness that substance abuse disorders often co-occur with major psychiatric disorders is growing. Abrams and Teplin (15) found that 59 percent of the inmates in the Cook County jail who had a diagnosis of schizophrenia also had a current alcohol abuse disorder, and 42 percent had a current drug dependence disorder.

Case managers for potentially violent clients with substance abuse problems should actively and aggressively pursue substance abuse treatment for their clients. In addition, as case managers develop trusting relationships with clients, case managers should reinforce that staying away from alcohol and illegal drugs will increase clients' chances of remaining in the community.

Cultural issues. Traditional mental health programs are staffed by credentialed mental health professionals who are typically white and middle-class. However, clients who are likely to be arrested generally do not share this demographic profile and may have opted not to use traditional mental health services because they feel disenfranchised. Many variables that influence the development of violence and crime among people with mental illness in the community may also contribute to their poverty, low levels of education, and underemployment.

To increase the relevance of case management services to these clients, mental health systems should try to employ case managers who are culturally similar to the clients they serve. In our opinion, cultural similarity may be more important than an advanced degree in one of the mental health professions in preparing the case manager to serve high-risk clients.

Cultural issues may include a variety of factors in addition to race and ethnicity. For example, clients with a hearing impairment typically grow up in a subculture quite different from that of persons without such impairments. Clients who are homosexual may need a different array of social supports than heterosexual clients. Persons who are arrested while passing through an area will require linkages with different types of services than will lifelong residents.

Human resources. Intensive case managers tend to have particular characteristics that distinguish them

The best intensive care managers for clients at high risk of becoming violent are those who have prior experience in a variety of service locations in both the mental health and criminal justice systems.

from staff of typical mental health programs. They should be creative, self-directed, independent people with little need for formal structure. Clearly, this work is not for everyone. In our experience, the most crucial element is experience, not formal education.

The best intensive case managers for clients at high risk of becoming violent are those who have prior experience in a variety of service locations in both the mental health and criminal justice systems. Former police officers may be particularly appropriate candidates for this job. Many police officers and others who work in the criminal justice system view themselves primarily as human service professionals. Their work involves supervising and supporting individuals, besides enforcing the law. Many police officers have a college degree when they begin police work or obtain a degree during their police career. They typically retire after 20 or 25 years of police service and thus constitute a potential cadre of experienced, yet young, service professionals with strong linkages with the criminal justice system.

Another group of potential intensive case managers are people who have succeeded in gaining control of their life circumstances despite their own serious mental illnesses (16). In addition to having developed networks of peer support, knowledge of responsive treatment providers, and strategies for meeting various needs, people who have been treated for mental illness may also be perceived as more credible sources of information by their prospective clients. More generally, case managers of every background can benefit from the insights and support of the emerging self-help movement of mental health service recipients (17).

Case management is a stressful business. Clients who are not cooperative can be frightening and a source of frustration to case managers. Yet if such clients form a bond with a case manager, the relationship may become intensely dependent and leave the case manager feeling drained. Case managers' salaries are typically low, and case managers are unlikely to receive benefits enjoyed by law enforcement officials, such as retirement after 20 years.

Further, case managers may feel that they are in personal danger, especially if they work with clients who have been violent in the past or if their work includes visiting the high-crime areas where many people with serious mental illness live. Case managers must frequently provide coverage after usual working hours, which can put a strain on their health as well as on their relationships. Finally, case managers may not have the prospect of upward career mobility. All of these factors lead to job stress and a high turnover rate. Administrators should thus pay attention to the need for ongoing training and support of case managers.

Conclusions

The keys to reducing the risk of violence by persons with mental disorder in the community are aggressive case management and a comprehensive array of support services. Although some specialized clinical services aimed at reducing violence per se may be needed, most of the services required by this client population are those that any person with serious mental disorder needs. The crucial difference is the increased intensity of case management for potentially violent clients.

Intensive case management for potentially violent clients requires case managers with special skills and low caseloads. The case managers must truly be "boundary spanners" (18) who understand and are able to negotiate the medical care, social service, housing assistance, and criminal justice systems as well as the mental health system.

This special kind of case manager does exist. We have seen them in many intensive case management and jail diversion programs throughout the U.S. They know what kinds of services are available and how to help their clients gain access to them. If clients drop out of a treatment program, intensive case managers attempt to find them and reconnect them to the services they need. If clients are arrested, intensive case managers do not drop them from their caseloads but continue working for them.

Intensive case management is not a panacea. It will fail if appropriate treatment and human services are not available in the community. As Goldman and colleagues (19) observed, the brokering and linkage roles of case management mean little if services are not available in the community to be brokered or linked. Case management may be but one piece of a comprehensive mental health care system, but it is the key to managing the risk of violence in the community among people with mental illness. ♦

References

1. Oliver C: "Wild man" puts fear in folks on Upper West Side. New York Post, Aug 26, 1992
2. Dugger CW: Threat only when on crack, homeless man foils system. New York Times, Sept 3, 1992
3. Shapiro E: Fear returns to sidewalks of West 96th Street along with homeless man. New York Times, Aug 26, 1992
4. Bachrach LL: Case management revisited. Hospital and Community Psychiatry 43:209–210, 1992
5. Solomon P: The efficacy of case management of services for severely mentally disabled clients. Community Mental Health Journal 28:163–180, 1992
6. Rubin A: Is case management effective for people with serious mental illness? A research review. Health and Social Work 17:138–150, 1992
7. Surles RC, Blanch AK, Shern DL, et al: Case management as a strategy for systems change. Health Affairs 11:151–163, 1992
8. Stein LI: On the abolishment of the case manager. Health Affairs 11:172–177, 1992
9. Bachrach LL: Young adult chronic patients: an analytical review of the literature. Hospital and Community Psychiatry 33:189–197, 1982
10. Massaro RP: The impact of physical health problems on psychiatric rehabilitation technology. Psychosocial Rehabilitation Journal 15:113–117, 1992
11. Sheila A, Joseph GR, Felton H, et al: Adult Intensive Case Management Evaluation. Albany, New York State Office of Mental Health, June 30, 1992
12. Wilson D, Tien G, Eaves D: An Assertive Case Management Program for Mentally Disordered Offenders: The Inter-Ministerial Project. Burnaby, British Columbia, Forensic Psychiatric Services, undated
13. Nancy H: Project Action: program evaluation. Presented at a Solutions 2000 conference, Houston, Sept 30, 1992
14. Peters RW, Hill HA: Inmates with co-occurring substance abuse and mental health disorders, in Mental Illness in America's Prisons. Edited by Steadman HJ, Cocozza JJ. Seattle, National Coalition for the Mentally Ill in the Criminal Justice System, 1993
15. Abrams KM, Teplin LA: Co-occurring disorders among jail detainees: implications for public policy. American Psychologist 46:1036–1045, 1991
16. Nikkel RE, Smith G, Edwards D: A consumer-operated case management project. Hospital and Community Psychiatry 43:577–579, 1992
17. Chamberlain J, Rogers J, Sneed C: Consumers, families, and community support systems. Psychosocial Rehabilitation Journal 14:83–85, 1989
18. Steadman HJ: Boundary spanners: a key component for the effective interactions of the justice and mental health systems. Law and Human Behavior 16:75–87, 1992
19. Goldman HH, Morrissey JP, Ridgely MS, et al: Lessons from the program on chronic mental illness. Health Affairs 11:51–68, 1992

Pharmacological and Behavioral Treatments for Aggressive Psychiatric Inpatients

Patrick W. Corrigan, Psy.D.
Stuart C. Yudofsky, M.D.
Jonathan M. Silver, M.D.

Aggressive behaviors of psychiatric patients may be caused by biological factors, environmental contingencies, or interactions thereof. Treatment teams are therefore best prepared to deal with these incidents when their armamentaria include a wide range of interventions.

Unfortunately, drug therapies have been traditionally promoted for remediation of "biological" symptoms, and behavioral treatments have been proffered for amelioration of "acquired" aggression, with the two approaches making mutually exclusive claims. A multidimensional approach to aggression assumes an interaction between biological and environmental etiologies as well as between drug and behavioral treatments.

In this paper, strategies in each domain of intervention are reviewed. Based on research findings, a decision tree for planning appropriate interventions with these patients is presented.

Frequency and consequences
Physical assault and property destruction rank among the most severe patient behaviors, frequently creating major treatment problems in inpatient settings. For example, 7 percent of patients in the psychiatric institutions of New York State committed at least one assault in a three-month period (1). Similarly, 12,000 assaults occurred in

Objective: Because aggressive behaviors of psychiatric patients may be caused by environmental or biological factors, treatment plans that incorporate medication and behavior therapies are the most effective. The authors review research on pharmacological and behavioral treatments for aggressive patients and present a decision tree for use on behavioral units to direct treatment of such patients. *Methods:* The empirical literature was searched for studies of pharmacological and behavioral interventions that have been shown to have some value for treating this problem. *Results and conclusions:* Psychiatrists must proceed cautiously because no medication has been approved by the Food and Drug Administration specifically for treatment of aggression. Antipsychotics, lithium, antidepressants, sedatives, anxiolytics, anticonvulsants, opiate antagonists, and beta blockers have been used, often depending on the etiology of the aggression, such as head injury or dementia. Although some drugs such as buspirone and propranolol show promise, side effects must be monitored. Three behavioral strategies have effectively reduced aggression in the inpatient milieu. The token economy is perhaps the most comprehensive behavioral tool for producing a well-structured milieu. Aggression replacement strategies help patients learn alternative responses. Decelerative techniques teach strategies that enable the patient to reduce aggression quickly. The authors describe a decision tree to guide decisions about pharmacological and behavioral treatments of aggression depending on where in the course of the disorder patients exhibit difficulty.

When this paper was published Dr. Corrigan was assistant professor of clinical psychiatry in the department of psychiatry at Pritzker School of Medicine of the University of Chicago. Dr. Yudofsky was professor of psychiatry at Baylor University School of Medicine in Houston. Dr. Silver was assistant professor of psychiatry at Columbia University College of Physicians and Surgeons in New York City. From the February 1993 issue of Hospital and Community Psychiatry (volume 44, pages 125–133).

all New York State institutions in a 12-month period (2). Violent behavior is not limited to young or psychotic patients; relatively high incidence rates have been found in geriatric (3,4) and developmentally disabled (5,6) samples.

Aggressive episodes significantly affect hostile patients and their treatment milieu. They may be injured when flailing against physical objects or hurt while being restrained by clinical staff or security personnel. Often staff and other patients are injured while in the vicinity of violent altercations or while trying to help restrain assaultive patients (7–9). Furthermore, frequent threats, personal violence, and property destruction undermine ward morale. Patients and clinicians alike become fearful of future physical outbursts and may withdraw from peers and staff on the unit (10–12). Seclusion and restraint are traditional aggression management methods used to protect inpatients and milieu staff from harm.

Unfortunately, seclusion and restraint present therapeutic and ethical problems. These procedures frequently require physical force, which increases the risk of patient or staff injury. Often seclusion and restraint do not teach patients coping skills that will help them avoid future aggression. Use of seclusion fosters distrust and dislike between patients and staff, which is contrary to most clinicians' professional philosophies. Appropriate psychopharmacological and behavioral interventions provide a potent means of avoiding the reactive use of seclusion and restraint.

Assessment

The first step in management of aggressive episodes entails identifying the biological and environmental precipitants of violent behavior. Five criteria that distinguish aggressive episodes with biological etiology from those that are principally environmental in origin have been identified (13,14). First, for patients whose aggression is biologically caused, historical data, neuropsychological test scores, or results of neurological examinations will likely provide evidence of central nervous system lesions or dysfunctions. Second, organically based incidents are sudden and relatively unprovoked. Third, violent outbursts of patients with biologically based aggression are relatively less controlled. Fourth, organically based incidents are well demarcated; patients seem to move from calm to rage to calm quickly. Finally, patients with biologically based rage typically show remorse.

Both self-report and observation-based instruments have been developed to describe the frequency and quality of assaults and to help differentiate biological from environmental precipitants. Self-report measures of aggression include the Buss-Durkee Hostility Inventory (15) and Novaco's measure (16) of anger and aggression. In addition, subscales of other measures, for example, the Brief Psychiatric Rating Scale (17), include items that address aggression and hostility.

Unfortunately, self-report inventories of aggression are limited by patients' insight into their problems and their willingness to admit to behavior of which most people disapprove. For example, one study found no correlation between scores on the Buss-Durkee inventory and observed aggression (18). The Nurses' Observation Scale for Inpatient Evaluation (NOSIE) avoids many of the pitfalls of self-report measures, because staff observe and rate patient violence (19). Unfortunately, the NOSIE is limited in range of test items and sensitivity to aggression.

As an alternative, the Overt Aggression Scale (OAS) was developed as an observation-based measure of verbal and physical aggression that can be easily completed by staff or family (20–22). The OAS comprises four items that assess verbal and physical aggression against self, objects, or others. It has been shown to have good interrater reliability (21), to correlate with independent ratings of aggression (20), and to correlate with severity of staff reaction (22). Single-case research strategies also provide an observation-based technology for monitoring the effects of psychopharmacological and behavioral treatments (23).

Psychopharmacological interventions

At this time no medication has been approved by the Food and Drug Administration specifically for treatment of aggression. Therefore, psychiatrists must act cautiously when using drugs to treat violent behavior. Several classes of psychotropic medication—antipsychotics, lithium, antidepressants, sedatives, buspirone, anticonvulsants, and beta blockers—have been clinically and experimentally tested on aggressive patients. Findings from this literature, summarized in Table 1, may guide clinical decisions about type and dose of drug.

Antipsychotics. Antipsychotics have been the most commonly used drugs for the treatment of aggression. A literature search of the efficacy of different drugs for aggression showed that antipsychotics were usually the first prescribed (24). Typically, the sedative effects rather than the antipsychotic properties of neuroleptics diminish aggression. Prolonged sedation, however, seriously diminishes patients' quality of life and essentially places the patients in chemical restraints.

Ironically, extended use of antipsychotic medication may exacerbate dyscontrol, rage, and violence. A double-blind study of 51 developmentally disabled subjects demonstrated that thioridazine led to an increase in aggressive and hostile behavior (25). While antipsychotic medication is usually helpful when aggression results from acute psychoses (such as violent responses to delusional threats), use of neuroleptic agents to treat chronic aggression—especially episodes that are caused by brain injury—is often ineffective and may result in debilitating side effects.

Lithium. Studies have shown lithium to be effective in the treatment of aggression secondary to mania; however, research has also suggested that lithium may effectively diminish hostile behaviors resulting from other biological etiologies (24). Case reports, open clinical trials, and double-blind, placebo-controlled studies have indicated that lithium significantly decreases the aggressive acts of mentally retarded patients. Similarly, empirical investigations of the effects of lithium on children with behavior disorders, head-injured adults, prison inmates, schizophrenic adults, or adults with personality disorders found that lithium significantly diminished aggression and self-injurious behavior. Paradoxically, other findings have suggested that lithium increases the frequency of aggressive behaviors in patients with temporal lobe epilepsy (26).

Unfortunately, outcomes of many of these studies were confounded by methodological flaws such as lack of a double-blind, placebo-controlled study design and vague methods of quantifying aggressive events. Until questions about the efficacy and specificity of lithium's effects are resolved, clinicians should consider limiting use of lithium to patients whose aggression is related to mania or to recurrent irritability associated with cyclic affective disorders.

Antidepressants. Several reports have described the use of antidepressants to control aggressive behavior associated with mood changes. These medications have their effects mainly in the serotonergic system, which has been shown to have an important role in the modulation of impulsive and aggressive behavior in several clinical populations (27). For example, in open studies, amitriptyline was shown to be effective in the treatment of patients with severe brain injury whose agitation had not responded to behavioral techniques (28-30). Trazodone has also been reported effective in treating aggression that occurs with organic mental disorders (31,32).

Sedatives. This category of medication includes the benzodiazepines, barbiturates, and related drugs such as chloral hydrate and paraldehyde. In the short term, the greatest effects of these drugs on aggression is the sedation of patients who are currently assaultive and who are unresponsive to verbal commands or gentle physical guidance.

However, prolonged use of high doses of benzodiazepines may result in confusion, dependency, or exacerbation of concomitant depression. Moreover, research has shown that prolonged administration of benzodiazepines may create a disinhibiting effect so that patients' aggression actually increases (33-35). Other reports have indicated that paradoxical agitation after treatment with benzodiazepines is uncommon (36). Thus we recommend use of these drugs during periods of current assaultive

Table 1
Psychopharmacological treatment of aggression[1]

Agent	Indications	Special considerations
Antipsychotics	Aggression directly related to psychotic ideation; acute management of violence or aggression using sedative side effects	Oversedation and multiple side effects including risk of tardive dyskinesia when used to treat chronic aggression
Lithium	Aggression and irritability related to mania	May be effective in prison populations or with mentally retarded patients
Antidepressants	Alternate drug for treating mood-related aggression	Significant effects on many patient populations with mood disorders
Sedatives	Acute management of violence or agitation using sedative and and hypnotic properties	Possible induction of paradoxical rage; problems with oversedation
Buspirone	Aggression related to anxiety	New research on effects; no negative findings yet
Anticonvulsants	Aggression related to complex seizure disorder; possibly aggression related to other organic brain disorders	Monitor patient closely for evidence of bone marrow suppression or hematologic abnormalities
Opiate agonists	Self-injurious behavior	Especially effective with developmentally disabled patients
Beta blockers	Chronic or recurrent aggression in patients with organic brain diseases or injuries; chronic or recurrent aggression or irritability in patients whose aggression is not directly related to psychotic ideation	Latency period before onset of action may be four to six weeks

[1] Yudofsky and associates (24)

outbursts, not on an ongoing basis nor with patients who have exhibited chronic aggression.

Buspirone. In some cases, aggression covaries with anxiety in such a way that anxiolytics like buspirone decrease the manifestation of hostile behaviors. Clinical investigators have only recently begun to evaluate the efficacy of this drug for aggression management. In preliminary reports, buspirone, a serotonergic agonist, has been reported to be effective in the management of aggression and agitation in patients with head injury, dementia, and developmental disability (24). If findings continue to be positive, buspirone should be considered for patients whose agitated and aggressive behaviors are compounded by anxiety and depression.

Anticonvulsants. Several studies have shown that the aggressive behaviors of psychiatric patients, especially those with abnormal electroencephalograms (EEGs), significantly diminished after administration of carbamazepine (37-39). In one study, aggressive behaviors of eight schizophrenic patients who were refractory to neuroleptic medication diminished significantly after a course of carbamazepine (40). The EEGs of all patients in this group showed generalized slowing. Several open studies have indicated that carbamazepine may be effective in decreasing hostile behavior associated with dementia (41,42). Despite the significant effects of carbamazepine, the clinician must beware of the potential effects of this medication, particularly bone marrow suppression (including aplastic anemia) and hepatotoxicity.

Opiate antagonists. Several case reports (43–45) and open clinical trials (46) suggest that the opiate antagonist naltrexone reduces self-injurious behavior. This effect is particularly notable in patients with developmental disabilities. A review by Konicki and Schulz (47) presents a detailed discussion of this topic.

Beta blockers. The effects of propranolol on aggressive behaviors of child and adult psychiatric patients have been demonstrated in several case studies and open clinical trials (24). In perhaps the best-controlled investigation of this kind, ten aggressive patients with organic brain disease participated in a randomized, double-blind, placebo-controlled, crossover study of propranolol (48). Before the study, these subjects had demonstrated little anger reduction after trials of antipsychotics, antidepressants, minor tranquilizers, or lithium. Results of the study showed that seven of the patients demonstrated moderate or marked improvement, two showed no improvement, and one patient dropped out because of medication side effects. Reports on other beta blockers like nadolol, pindolol, and metoprolol have shown that they diminish aggression as well. Several side effects have been identified and include hypotension, bradycardia, and in rare cases depression (49). Detailed guidelines for administering and monitoring propranolol have been outlined elsewhere (24).

Behavioral interventions

In inpatient behavioral programs, the form of the staff-patient relationship is highly prescribed so that frustrating and potentially violent altercations resulting from confusing interactions are decreased. The well-structured milieu decreases violent episodes by fostering more socially appropriate responses among patients; patients with these skills are less in need of responding aggressively (50).

The token economy

The token economy is perhaps the most comprehensive behavioral tool for producing a well-structured milieu (51–53). Three steps must be completed to implement a token economy. First, interpersonal and self-care behaviors that can be increased by a token economy are identified, and methods for increasing them are outlined. Second, contingencies that specify the number of tokens received for each target behavior are constructed. Contingencies describe if-then relationships between response and consequence that differ for different behaviors and different patients. For example, if Ms. B, who rarely washes herself, bathes before 8 a.m., then she will receive four tokens. The third step in implementing a token economy is to post rules for token exchange. For example, patients are informed that the token store is open at 9 a.m. each day and that they can buy a cup of juice for three tokens.

Reinforcing patients' prosocial behaviors can proactively decrease the level of hostility and aggression on the inpatient unit. Response costs (54) are typically used in token economies to reactively reduce aggression. Patients with mildly violent behaviors are fined a small number of tokens. Research has shown that inpatient units that have implemented token economies have significantly fewer aggressive episodes than more traditional settings (53).

Token economies are institutionalized systems for contingency management. Unitwide behaviors and consequences that apply to all patients are identified, and information about them is disseminated. Idiosyncratic behaviors that are missed by token economies can be specifically targeted using a behavioral contract (55). Behavioral contracts are also if-then assertions that include a statement of the behavior and a consequence: "If you do not yell at your roommate today, then you can have a grounds pass after dinner." The worth of the contract is determined by whether the targeted behavior increases.

Other behavioral strategies may be incorporated into inpatient programs to diminish aggressive incidents. Such strategies can be clustered into two groups, including aggression replacement strategies that help patients acquire response alternatives to aggression and decelerative techniques that teach strategies by which the patient is able to reduce aggression quickly (56–58).

Aggression replacement

Careful observation within the behavioral milieu may identify previolent behaviors that precede assault or property destruction (59). Previolent behaviors include obvious signs such as yelling, swearing, or threatening, as well as more subtle verbal and nonverbal messages. Aggression can be better managed when staff establish contingencies that diminish the frequency of previolent behaviors and help patients learn social and coping skills to replace these behaviors. Replacement methods include manipulating rewards and punishments that maintain aggressive behaviors and teaching patients behavioral alternatives to assaultive responses. Specific strategies are summarized in Table 2.

Reinforcement strategies are most effective when treatment planners select stimuli that are known to be rewarding for an individual patient. This approach requires a thorough survey of the patient's reinforcement history plus careful observation of the environmental rewards that are effective.

Differential reinforcement schedules. Laboratory research shows that when responses other than inappropriate target behavior are reinforced on an intensive schedule, frequency of the target behavior decreases (60,61). When using differential reinforcement of other behavior for decreasing agitation, staff reinforce all behaviors except the aggressive target. For example, using such a strategy, staff rewarded Mr. J—a particularly loud and angry patient—for sitting quietly and talking pleasantly during waking hours; in short, he was rewarded for everything other than yelling. The frequency and size of payoff for specific differential reinforcement schedules depend on the severity of the target behavior. Because Mr. J was yelling several times each day, he received five tokens for every ten minutes that he was not hostile. As the target decreases in frequency, payoff diminishes.

Though effective, such schedules are extremely resource intensive, requiring staff to be constantly vigilant for behaviors other than the target behavior and to pay out large number of tokens as reinforcers.

Differential reinforcement of incompatible behavior is a less intensive schedule that reinforces behaviors that inhibit or otherwise interfere with the performance of the target behavior. In our example, staff gave Mr. J tokens each time he controlled his anger by removing himself from frustrating situations or each time he made an assertive comment rather than a threat.

Assertiveness training. Occasionally, interpersonal frustrations escalate to aggressive responses because patients have not mastered assertive behaviors. Assertive behavior is a generic interpersonal skill that includes saying no, making a complaint, and expressing appreciation. Patients with few assertive skills can learn to say no and make complaints by participating in structured, psychoeducational modules (62–64). During these modules, patients watch staff demonstrate specific skills; patients then role play the skill. Trainers prompt patients on appropriate responses when they get stuck and provide feedback on the quality of patients' performance. Homework is assigned to patients to foster generalization of skills to settings outside the training milieu.

Patients armed with assertiveness skills will be better prepared to deal with future frustrations. Research has shown that patients with severe mental illness who participate in skills training programs demonstrate fewer psychotic symptoms (65,66) and increase their repertoire of interpersonal skills (67–70). Aggressive behaviors will probably diminish as patients' repertoire of social skills increases.

Activity programming in a tranquil milieu. Violent behaviors are more likely to occur when patients reside in a poorly structured milieu with undefined program rules and excessive unscheduled time. Research has shown that residential units that are visually or aurally overstimulating may exacerbate psychosis (71). Thus the treatment setting must be structured by unit rules so that levels of sensory stimulation are moderate to low. To accomplish this goal, televisions, stereos, and musical instruments should be restricted to soundproofed areas. Lighting, temperature, wall colors, and air quality should not be provocative or overstimulating.

Inpatient units that provide a rich assortment of productive activities (for example, games, sports, reading, writing, group therapy, recreational outings, and occupational therapy) diminish the likelihood of inappropriate behavior. Structured, supervised activities have been used to reduce inappropriate behavior and increase adaptive social, leisure, and instrumental functioning (Corrigan PW, Liberman RP, Wong S, unpublished study, 1991). In settings like these, activities are scheduled five days a week, during which time ward staff verbally prompt patients to engage in independent or group activities. These activity periods constitute behavioral settings that provide patients with strong cues about expectations for appropriate and inappropriate behavior, rules and goals of the setting, and roles of individuals in the setting. The interactional rules and intrinsic rewards available in structured activities result in fewer assaultive episodes and less disorganized behavior (72–75).

Decelerative techniques

Even when aggression replacement strategies have increased patients' prosocial, nonhostile behaviors, assaultive incidents may still occur on

Table 2

Behavioral treatment of aggression

Strategy	Indications	Special considerations
Token economy	Provides both proactive and reactive strategies for aggressive behaviors	A structured format for implementing contingency management
Aggression replacement		
Differential reinforcement schedules	Replaces punishing contingency for previolent behavior	Differential reinforcement of other behaviors is resource intensive; differential reinforcement of incompatible behaviors requires identification of suitable interfering behaviors
Assertiveness training	Effective for patients who become angry when their needs are not met	Patients must work well in skills training groups
Activity programming	Diminishes opportunities for unstructured, frustrating interactions	Activities that patients find reinforcing should be identified
Decelerative techniques		
Social extinction	Effective with previolent patients who respond to social reinforcements	May not work with schizoid patients
Contingent observation	Effective with previolent patients who respond to social reinforcements	Patients must be sufficiently organized to accurately perceive models
Self-controlled time out	Effective with violent patients immediately after incidents	May diminish risky attempts to seclude or restrain
Overcorrection	Effective with relatively docile patients	Stop if patient struggles with guided practice
Contingent restraint	Effective with violent patients who do not comply with self-controlled time out and are resistant to guided practice	Decreases inadvertent reinforcement of behaviors that covary with seclusion and restraint

behavioral units. Behavior therapy provides a hierarchy of intervention strategies that may stop assaults, remove secondary gains, and, in some instances, provide learning opportunities for patients to acquire alternative responses. These strategies are summarized in hierarchical order in Table 2.

Responses in the hierarchy are ranked from least intrusive—involving minimal humiliation or risk of physical injury—to most intrusive, involving higher risk of injury. Staff on inpatient units must establish criteria for implementing various levels of restriction. Clinicians should select interventions that are least restrictive and most empirically effective. Decisions about what interventions best meet these criteria are facilitated by having available a comprehensive history of each patient's problem and reactions to past interventions.

Decelerative techniques are punitive in nature and therefore are likely to quickly reduce the frequency of targeted behaviors. These decrements, however, will be maintained only if the techniques are paired with reinforcing strategies that teach patients coping skills.

Social extinction. Many patients like to talk with staff members. Thus withdrawal of staff attention when these patients exhibit aggressive behaviors may decrease the rate of future aggression, especially if evidence suggests that violent outbursts are maintained by attention from peers or staff. Extinction is most commonly used with mildly aggressive or disruptive behaviors that do not require immediate staff response (for example, threatening gestures or loud vocalizations). Staff explicitly define the target behavior and the amount of time they will ignore the patient in an effort to extinguish the behavior. Effective extinction requires all staff to ignore the designated patient during the intervention. Thus staff should not discuss the inappropriate behavior with the patient and should avoid eye contact. Staff who were not present when the inappropriate behavior was exhibited should be notified that an extinction schedule has been implemented so that they interact with the patient in a manner consistent with other clinicians.

B. F. Skinner (76) found in his research with laboratory animals that immediately before a target behavior was extinguished, it increased in frequency. Thus one would expect assaultive behaviors that are being extinguished by staff to initially become more severe. For example, inpatient staff who were ignoring Mr. J's loud voice noted that the frequency of thunderous comments actually increased soon after the strategy was implemented. Staff need to be educated on this point so that they do not prematurely relinquish the intervention strategy. If used consistently, extinction may be an effective means to diminish the rate of inappropriate behaviors (77).

Contingent observation. While social extinction may remove subtle interpersonal behaviors that maintain previolent behaviors, it does not include a learning opportunity by which patients can acquire replacement behaviors. In response to previolent behaviors, clinicians using contingent observation instruct acting-out patients to sit quietly for a predefined time on the perimeter of the group (78). While sitting alone, patients are instructed to watch peers and staff carefully and observe alternative responses they might use to avoid future angry responses. Staff verbally reinforce patients when they are quietly watching others. The observation period continues until patients remain calm for two minutes, at which time they may return to the group.

Self-controlled time out. Time out from reinforcement is an operant technique in which socially inappropriate behaviors can be decreased by short-term removal of patients from overstimulating (and perhaps reinforcing) situations. Time out is most effective with patients who experience loss of social contact as punitive. Unlike seclusion, however, self-controlled time out provokes less reaction because patients have some control over the process. In this way, time out offers a less restrictive alternative to seclusion and restraint, engenders less humiliation, and involves less risk of injury.

Patients who perform aggressive acts are prompted to enter time out, usually one corner of a quiet, low-traffic room, and to remain in the quiet area until they have been nonaggressive for two minutes. Sometimes a patient's continued aggression in the time-out area may result in a lengthy intervention. However, time-out periods that are excessive become overly punitive and diminish the effect of the intervention. Patients who do not comply with time-out instructions after one minute are told to enter the seclusion room. Thus seclusion is used as a punishment for patients who do not comply with the time-out prompt. Research on self-controlled time out has shown that use of this technique significantly diminished the number of dangerous interactions involving seclusion or restraint on a unit for treatment-refractory patients (79).

Overcorrection. Overcorrection uses the time-out strategy and also requires the patient to reduce the rate of offensive behaviors by forcefully replacing them with more prosocial alternatives (80–83). The requirement compels patients to restore the disturbed situation to a vastly improved condition. For example, a patient who hits someone might be required to apologize to the victim, the other patients on the ward, and the staff.

Frequently, gentle force may be necessary to guide the patient to begin the task. A patient who throws soda in the day room may be physically guided to pick up a sponge and wash the wall thoroughly. Only the minimum force necessary to implement the overcorrection procedure should be used. Although manual guidance may at first be necessary to establish instructional control, the procedure is contraindicated for patients who repeatedly refuse to participate after the initial guidance period. Extreme caution with this approach is warranted; any coercive program applied to recalcitrant patients may escalate into incidents of staff injury or patient abuse.

Contingent restraint. Contingent restraint is operationally similar to conventional restraining methods; however, it demands immediate and consistent administration of restraint after each episode of severe violence.

Figure 1

Decision tree for selecting intervention strategies for aggressive patients, based on biological and environmental factors

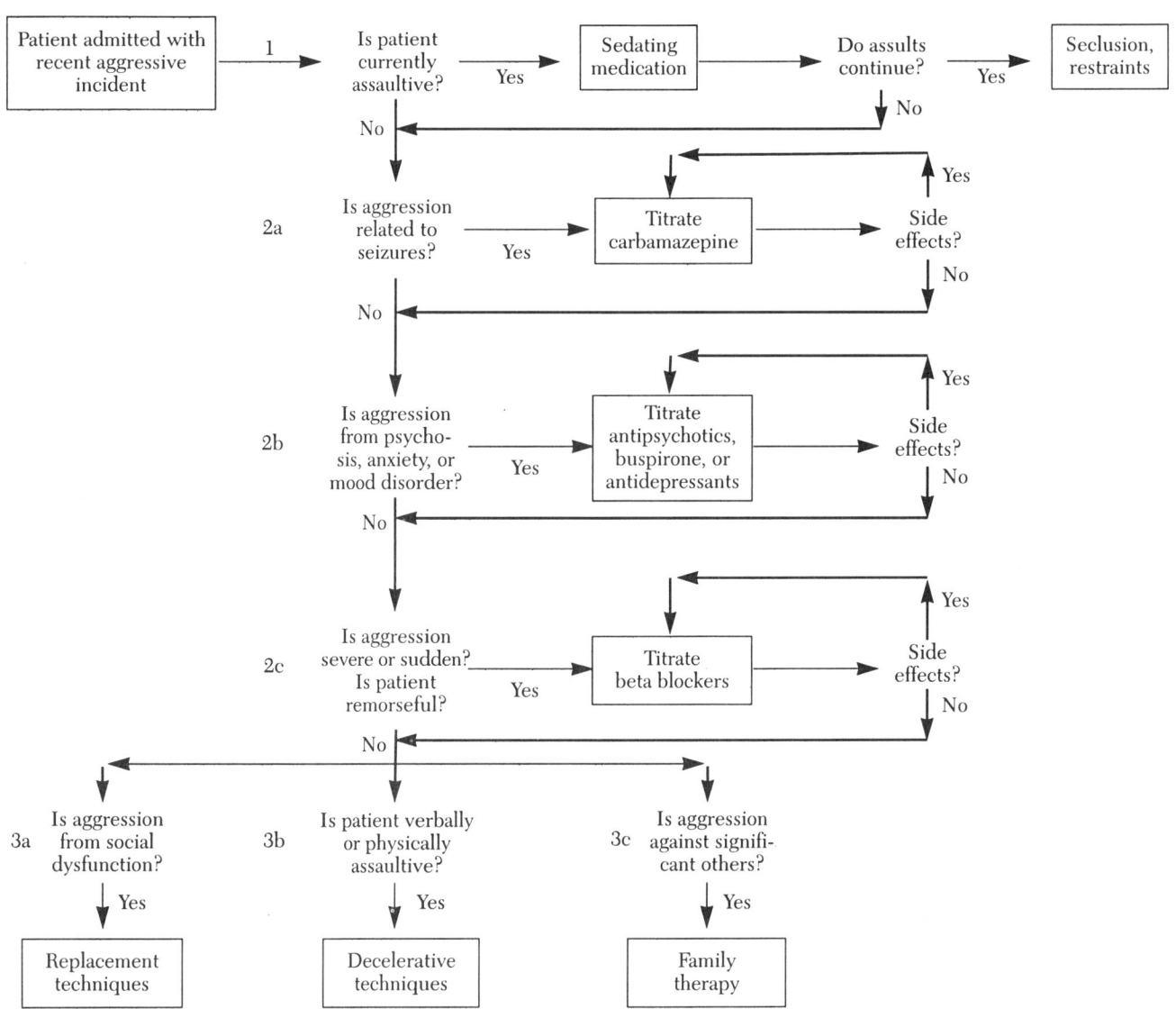

Moreover, staff do not interact verbally with patients during restraints so as not to reinforce the maladaptive behavior inadvertently. Clinicians should be wary of patients who sleep while in restraints or otherwise appear to enjoy being restrained (84,85).

Interactive application of interventions

Figure 1 outlines a decision tree that can guide the informed clinician through comprehensive evaluation and treatment of aggressive inpatients. Treatment occurs in a behavioral milieu that uses aggression replacement strategies. Decisions are based on the three sets of numbered questions. Is the patient currently assaultive? What are the biological precipitants of aggression? What are the environmental precipitants?

Although this arrangement of questions presumes that the decision-making process is hierarchical, we are not implying that options either within or across decision sets should be rigidly considered. In particular, knowledge about therapeutic benefits and side effects of psychotropic medication for aggression is continually evolving. The full range of symptoms and behaviors needs to be monitored to ensure that untoward consequences of medication are quickly addressed.

The first step after admission is to determine whether the patient is currently assaultive and whether the assaults represent a risk to patients and staff. For a patient judged to be a present danger, clinicians must weigh the relative costs and benefits of sedative medications versus seclusion or restraint in subduing a physically violent person. During this stage, assessment of the biological precipitants of patient aggression begins as well; identification and treatment of these precipitants reduce the time during which sedation or seclusion is required.

The decision about physiological precipitants is arranged hierarchically. For example, aggressive patients who show evidence of a seizure disorder might receive carbamazepine first. Patients with psychotic symptoms might be considered for relatively high doses of neuroleptics to handle acute episodes. Patients whose aggression does not remit and who show mood-congruent or anxiety-related agitation might be evaluated for either antidepressant or buspirone trials. In cases when aggression does not remit after antipsychotic or antiseizure medication regimens have been tried, or when aggression meets several of the signs of organically based aggression, beta blockers might be indicated.

The decision tree in Figure 1 assumes that the entire decision-making process occurs within a behavioral milieu that is fostering prosocial (and thus antiassaultive) interactions by using aggression replacement methods. Environmental precipitants of aggression may include never having learned appropriate social skills (in which case assertiveness skills training is indicated) or having acquired aggressive behaviors that were rewarded in other situations (in which case decelerative techniques are used). Sometimes components of aggression may be specific to or exacerbated by patients' families or other social networks. In these situations, significant others are trained in aggression replacement and decelerative methods to help generalize diminished aggression to situations outside the inpatient unit. ♦

References

1. Tardiff K, Sweillam A: Assault, suicide, and mental illness. Archives of General Psychiatry 73:164–169, 1982
2. New York State Senate Select Committee on Mental and Physical Handicap: Violence Revisited: A Report on Traditional Indifference in State Mental Institutions Toward Assaultive Activity. Albany, New York Senate, 1977
3. Chandler JD, Chandler JE: The prevalence of neuropsychiatric disorders in a nursing home population. Journal of Geriatric Psychiatry and Neurology 1:71–76, 1988
4. Evans DA, Funkenstein HH, Albert MS, et al: Prevalence of Alzheimer's disease in a community population of older persons. JAMA 262:2551–2556, 1989
5. Reid AH, Ballinger BR, Heather BB, et al: The natural history of behavioral symptoms among severely and profoundly mentally retarded patients. British Journal of Psychiatry 145:289–293, 1984
6. Rabins PV, Mace NL, Lukas MJ: The impact of dementia on the family. JAMA 248:333–335, 1982
7. Pearson M, Wilmot E, Padi M: A study of violent behaviour among in-patients in a psychiatric hospital. British Journal of Psychiatry 149:232–235, 1986
8. Lion JR, Snyder W, Merrill GL: Underreporting of assaults on staff in a state hospital. Hospital and Community Psychiatry 32:497–498, 1981
9. Madden DJ, Lion JR, Penna MW: Assaults on psychiatrists by patients. American Journal of Psychiatry 133:422–425, 1976
10. Klass DG, Growe A, Strizich M: Ward treatment milieu and posthospital functioning. Archives of General Psychiatry 34:1047–1052, 1977
11. Moos RH: Evaluating Treatment Environments: A Social Ecological Approach. New York, Wiley, 1974
12. Appelbaum PS: The new preventive detention: psychiatry's problematic responsibility for the control of violence. American Journal of Psychiatry 145:779–785, 1988
13. Yudofsky SC, Silver JM, Yudofsky B: Organic personality disorder, explosive type, in Treatment of Psychiatric Disorders. Edited by Karasu TB. Washington, DC, American Psychiatric Press, 1989
14. Yudofsky SC, Silver JM, Hales RE: Pharmacologic management of aggression in the elderly. Journal of Clinical Psychiatry 51(Oct suppl):22–28, 1990
15. Buss AH, Durkee A: An inventory for assessing different kinds of hostility. Journal of Consulting Psychology 21:343–349, 1957
16. Novaco RW: Anger Control: The Development and Evaluation of an Experimental Treatment. Lexington, Mass, Lexington Books, 1976
17. Lukoff D, Nuechterlein KH, Ventura J: Appendix A: manual for the expanded BPRS. Schizophrenia Bulletin 12:594–602, 1986
18. Edmunds G, Kendrick DC: The Measurement of Human Aggressiveness. Chichester, England, Ellis Horwood, 1980
19. Honigfeld G, Gillis RD, Klett CJ: Nurses' Observation Scale for Inpatient Evaluation: a new scale for measuring improvement in chronic schizophrenia. Journal of Clinical Psychology 21:65–71, 1965
20. Silver JM, Yudofsky SC: Documentation of aggression in the assessment of the violent patient. Psychiatric Annals 17:375–384, 1987
21. Silver JM, Yudofsky SC: The Overt Aggression Scale: overview and clinical guidelines. Journal of Neuropsychiatry and Clinical Neuroscience 3:197–212, 1991
22. Yudofsky SC, Silver JM, Jackson W, et al: The Overt Aggression Scale: an operationalized rating scale for verbal and physical aggression. American Journal of Psychiatry 143:35–39, 1986
23. Barlow DH, Hersen M: Single Case Experimental Designs: Strategies for Studying Behavior Change, 2nd ed. New York, Pergamon, 1984
24. Yudofsky SC, Silver JM, Schneider SE: Pharmacologic treatment of aggression. Psychiatric Annals 17:397–407, 1987
25. Elie R, Langlois Y, Cooper SF, et al: Comparison of SCH-12679 and thioridazine in aggressive mental retardates. Canadian Journal of Psychiatry 25:484–491, 1980
26. Schiff HB, Sabin TD, Geller A, et al: Lithium in aggressive behavior. American Journal of Psychiatry 138:1346–1348, 1982
27. Golden RN, Gilmore JH, Corrigan MHN, et al: Serotonin, suicide and aggression. Journal of Clinical Psychiatry 52(Dec suppl):61–69, 1991
28. Jackson RD, Corrigan JD, Arnett JA: Amitriptyline for agitation in head injury. Archives of Physical and Medical Rehabilitation 66:180–181, 1985
29. Mysiw WJ, Jackson RD, Corrigan JD: Amitriptyline for posttraumatic agitation. American Journal of Physical Medicine and Rehabilitation 2:29–33, 1988
30. Szlabowicz JW, Stewart JT: Amitriptyline treatment of agitation associated with anoxic encephalopathy. Archives of Physical Medicine and Rehabilitation 71:612–613, 1990
31. Greenwald BS, Marin DB, Silverman SM: Serotonergic treatment of screaming and banging in dementia. Lancet 2:1464–1465, 1986
32. Pinner E, Rich CL: Effects of trazodone on aggressive behavior in seven patients with organic mental disorders. American Journal of Psychiatry 145:1295–1296, 1988
33. Gardos G: Disinhibition of behavior by antianxiety drugs. Psychosomatics 21:1025–1026, 1980
34. Salzman C, Kochansky GE, Shader RI, et al: Chlordiazepoxide-induced hostility in a small group setting. Archives of General Psychiatry 31:401–405, 1974
35. Wilkinsin CJ: Effects of diazepam (Valium) and trait anxiety on human physical aggression and emotional state. Journal of Behavioral Medicine 8:101–115, 1985
36. Dietch JT, Jennings RK: Aggressive dyscontrol in patients treated with benzodiazepines. Journal of Clinical Psychiatry 49:184–189, 1988
37. Luchins DJ: Carbamazepine for the violent psychiatric patient (ltr). Lancet 1:766, 1983
38. Stone JL, McDaniel KD, Hughes JR, et al: Episodic dyscontrol disorder and proxymal EEG abnormalities: successful treatment with carbamazepine. Biological Psychiatry 21:208–212, 1986
39. Yatham LN, McHale PA: Carbamazepine in the treatment of aggression: a case report and review of the literature. Acta Psychiatrica Scandinavica 24:188–190, 1988
40. Hakoloa HP, Laulumaa VA: Carbamazepine in treatment of violent schizophrenics (ltr). Lancet 1:1358, 1982
41. Gleason RP, Schneider LS: Carbamazepine treatment of agitation in Alzheimer's outpatients refractory to neuroleptics. Journal of Clinical Psychiatry 51:115–118, 1990

42. Leibovici A, Tariot PN: Carbamazepine treatment of agitation associated with dementia. Journal of Geriatric Psychiatry and Neurology 1:110–112, 1988

43. Lienemann J, Walker P: Naltrexone for treatment of self-injury. American Journal of Psychiatry 146:1639–1640, 1989

44. Bernstein GA, Hughes JR, Mitchell JE, et al: Effects of narcotic antagonists on self-injurious behavior: a single case study. Journal of the American Academy of Child and Adolescent Psychiatry 26: 886–889, 1987

45. Richardson JG, Zaleski WA: Naloxone and self-mutilation. Biological Psychiatry 18: 99–101, 1983

46. Kars H, Broekma W, Glaudemans-van Gelderen I: Naltrexone attenuates self-injurious behavior in mentally retarded subjects. Biological Psychiatry 27:741–746, 1990

47. Konicki PE, Schulz C: Rationale for clinical trials of opiate antagonists in treating patients with personality disorders and self-injurious behavior. Psychopharmacology Bulletin 25:556–563, 1989

48. Greendyke RM, Schuster DB, Wooton JA: Propranolol in the treatment of assaultive patients with organic brain disease. Journal of Clinical Psychopharmacology 4:282–285, 1984

49. Paykel E, Fleminger R, Watson JP: Psychiatric aspects of hypertensive drugs other than reserpine. Journal of Clinical Psychopharmacology 2:14–39, 1982

50. Oldham JM, Russakoff LM, Prusnofsky L: Seclusion: patterns and milieu. Journal of Nervous and Mental Disease 171:645–650, 1983

51. Ayllon T, Azrin NH: The Token Economy: A Motivational System for Therapy and Rehabilitation. New York, Appleton-Century-Crofts, 1968

52. Kazdin AE: The token economy: a decade later. Journal of Applied Behavior Analysis 15:431–445, 1982

53. Paul GL, Lentz RJ: Psychosocial Treatment of the Chronic Mental Patient. Cambridge, Mass, Harvard University Press, 1977

54. Kazdin A: Response cost: the removal of conditioned reinforcers for therapeutic change. Behavior Therapy 3:533–546, 1972

55. DeRisi WJ, Butz G: Writing Behavioral Contracts: A Case Simulation Practice Manual. Champaign, Ill, Research Press, 1975

56. Lennox DB, Miltenberger RG, Sprengler P, et al: Decelerative treatment practices with persons who have mental retardation: a review of five years of the literature. American Journal of Mental Retardation 92:492–501, 1988

57. Liberman RP, Wong SE: Behavioral analysis and therapy procedures related to seclusion and restraint, in The Psychiatric Uses of Seclusion and Restraint. Edited by Tardiff K. Washington, DC, American Psychiatric Press, 1984

58. Corrigan PW, Liberman RP: Behavior therapy: an overview, in Behavior Therapy in Psychiatric Care. Edited by Corrigan PW, Liberman RP. New York, Springer, 1994

59. Kalogjera IJ, Bedi A, Watson WN, et al: Impact of therapeutic management on use of seclusion and restraint with disruptive adolescent inpatients. Hospital and Community Psychiatry 40:280–285, 1989

60. Homer AL, Peterson L: Differential reinforcement of other behavior: a preferred response elimination procedure. Behavior Therapy 11:449–471, 1980

61. Zeiler MD: Positive reinforcement and the elimination of reinforced responses. Journal of the Experimental Analysis of Behavior 26:37–44, 1976

62. Curran JP, Monti PM: (eds): Social Skills Training: A Practical Handbook for Assessment and Treatment. New York, Guilford, 1982

63. Lange AJ, Jakubowski P: Responsible Assertive Behavior: Cognitive/Behavioral Procedures for Trainers. Champaign, Ill, Research Press, 1976

64. Douglas MS, Mueser KT: Teaching conflict resolution skills to the chronically mentally ill: social skills training groups for briefly hospitalized patients. Behavior Modification 14:519–547, 1990

65. Hogarty GE, Anderson CM, Reiss DJ, et al: Family psychoeducation, social skills training, and maintenance chemotherapy in the aftercare treatment of schizophrenia. Archives of General Psychiatry 43:633–642, 1986

66. Liberman RP, Mueser KT, Wallace CJ: Social skills training for schizophrenic individuals at risk for relapse. American Journal of Psychiatry 143:523–526, 1986

67. Bellack AS, Turner SM, Hersen M, et al: An examination of the efficacy of social skills training for chronic schizophrenic patients. Hospital and Community Psychiatry 35:1023–1028, 1984

68. Brown MA, Munford AM: Life skills training for chronic schizophrenics. Journal of Nervous and Mental Disease 17:1466–1476, 1983

69. Hansen DJ, St Lawrence JS, Christoff KA: Effects of interpersonal problem-solving training with chronic aftercare patients on problem-solving component skills and effectiveness of solution. Journal of Consulting and Clinical Psychology 53:167–174, 1985

70. Van Dam-Baggen R, Kraaimmat F: A group social skills training program with psychiatric patients: outcome, dropout rate, and prediction. Behaviour Research and Therapy 34:161–169, 1986

71. Drake RE, Sederer LI: The adverse effects of intensive treatment of chronic schizophrenia. Comprehensive Psychiatry 27: 313–326, 1986

72. Wong SE, Terranova MD, Bowen L, et al: Providing independent recreational activities to reduce stereotypic verbalizations in chronic schizophrenics. Journal of Applied Behavioral Analysis 20:77–81, 1987

73. Wong SE, Wright J, Terranova MD, et al: Effects of structured ward activities on appropriate and psychotic behavior of chronic psychiatric patients. Behavioral Residential Treatment 3:41–50, 1988

74. Polsky RH, McGuire MT: Social ethology of acute psychiatric patients: the influence of sex, hospital environment, and spatial proximity. Journal of Nervous and Mental Disease 169:28–36, 1981

75. Rosen AJ, Sussman S, Mueser KT, et al: Behavioral assessment of psychiatric inpatients and normal controls across different environmental contexts. Journal of Behavioral Assessment 3:25–36, 1981

76. Skinner BF: Science of Human Behavior. New York, Macmillan, 1953

77. Liberman RP, Wallace CJ, Teigen J, et al: Interventions with psychotic behaviors, in Innovative Treatment Methods in Psychopathology. Edited by Calhoun KS, Adams HE, Mitchell KM. New York, Wiley, 1974

78. Porterfield JK, Herbert-Jackson E, Risley TR: Contingent observation: an effective and acceptable procedure for reducing disruptive behavior of young children in a group setting. Journal of Applied Behavior Analysis 9:55–64, 1976

79. Glynn SM, Bowen LL, Marshall BD, et al: Compliance with less restrictive aggression-control procedures. Hospital and Community Psychiatry 40:82–84, 1989

80. Foxx RM, Azrin NH: Restitution: a method of eliminating aggressive-disruptive behavior of retarded and brain damaged patients. Behavior Research and Therapy 10:15–27, 1972

81. Marholin DH, Luiselli JK, Townsend NM: Overcorrection: an examination of its rationale and treatment effectiveness, in Progress in Behavior Modification, vol 10. Edited by Hersen M, Eisler RM, Miller PM. New York, Academic Press, 1980

82. Ollendick TH, Matson JL: Overcorrection: an overview. Behavior Therapy 9:830–842, 1978

83. Sumner JH, Mueser ST, Hsu L, et al: Overcorrection treatment for radical reduction of aggressive-disruptive behavior in institutionalized mental patients. Psychological Reports 35:655–662, 1974

84. Favell E, McGimsey JF, Jones ML: The use of physical restraint in the treatment of self-injury and as a positive reinforcement. Journal of Applied Behavioral Analysis 11:225–241, 1978

85. Favell E, McGimsey JF, Jones ML, et al: Physical restraint as positive reinforcement. American Journal of Mental Deficiency 85:425–432, 1981

The Relationship Between Acute Psychiatric Symptoms, Diagnosis, and Short-Term Risk of Violence

Dale E. McNiel, Ph.D.
Renée L. Binder, M.D.

Clinicians are frequently required to assess the risk of violent behavior among persons with mental disorders in a variety of contexts (1–3). However, existing research has been of only limited benefit in providing an empirical base for evaluating the potential for violence among mentally ill persons.

Research with community samples has suggested that demographic variables such as age and gender are more important indicators of risk of violence than clinical variables such as diagnosis and symptoms (4), whereas studies with acutely disturbed patients evaluated shortly before or during hospitalization suggest that clinical variables are better predictors than demographic variables (5,6). Even in studies of acutely ill patients, the findings have been inconsistent. For example, although some studies have reported an overrepresentation of violent patients among specific diagnostic groups, such as schizophrenic patients, manic patients, and patients with organic brain syndromes (7–9), these conclusions have not been uniformly supported across other studies (10).

Findings that support a relationship between diagnosis and violence among acute patients suggest the potential utility of identifying features of acute illness that place patients at increased risk of violence. Some studies

Objective: Previous research on violence and mental disorder has typically focused on the relationship between diagnosis and risk of violence or between symptoms within a particular diagnostic category and risk of violence. The authors' goal was to evaluate whether the pattern of symptoms associated with short-term risk of violence varies depending on patients' diagnoses. *Methods:* Subjects were 330 patients with a variety of diagnoses who were hospitalized on a university-based, locked psychiatric inpatient unit. At hospital admission, physicians rated patients' symptoms using the Brief Psychiatric Rating Scale. Nurses rated whether patients became violent during hospitalization by completing the Overt Aggression Scale at the end of each shift. *Results:* Assaultive patients had different symptom patterns than nonassaultive patients. Symptom patterns varied significantly across diagnostic groups, and the symptom patterns associated with violence also varied significantly across diagnostic groups. Higher levels of hostile-suspiciousness, agitation-excitement, and thinking disturbance were generally associated with violence, although these symptoms were less predictive of assaultiveness among schizophrenic patients than among patients in other diagnostic groups. *Conclusions:* Symptom profiles represent a useful level of analysis for understanding the relationship between violence and psychopathology. However, the value of particular symptom profiles as indicators of imminent violence varies with diagnosis.

have reported associations between violence and symptoms such as hallucinations and delusions (11,12). Other studies have suggested that mental disorders such as schizophrenia or mania may each have distinctive symptom patterns that are associated with risk of violence (13,14). However, interpretation of these studies has been limited by methodological problems such as lack of control groups and use of dependent measures, such

---

When this paper was published Dr. McNiel *was an associate adjunct professor of psychology and* Dr. Binder *was professor in the department of psychiatry at the University of California, San Francisco. From the February 1994 issue of* Hospital and Community Psychiatry *(volume 45, pages 133–137).*

as incident reports, that underestimate the true rate of violence (15).

Previous studies that have assessed the relationship between symptoms and violence have not included control groups composed of patients with differing diagnoses. Because symptom patterns vary across diagnoses, the generalizability of findings from one diagnostic group, for example, schizophrenic patients, to other diagnostic groups, for example, manic patients, is unclear. Research providing this information could be important for identifying the specific aspects of mental disorder that indicate an increased probability of violence.

This study examines the relationship between acute psychopathology and short-term risk of violence in a sample of newly hospitalized acute patients. To our knowledge, this is the first study to evaluate whether the pattern of symptoms associated with short-term risk of violence varies depending on patients' diagnoses. We included control groups of patients with different diagnoses when evaluating the relationship between symptoms and short-term risk of violence. The relationship between diagnosis and risk of assault was also evaluated.

Methods

The study was conducted on a university-based, locked, short-term psychiatric inpatient unit with a mean length of stay of 18 days. In a previous study of symptoms and violence, data had been collected for 127 diagnostically heterogeneous patients admitted to the inpatient unit in 1988–1989 (16). For this study the sample was expanded to include an additional 203 patients who had been admitted to the unit between 1989 and 1990.

The two groups were combined, and their 330 medical records were reviewed for demographic data and primary diagnosis according to *ICD-9-CM*, the diagnostic system used by our hospital at the time of the study. By combining the two samples of patients, it was possible to obtain enough patients in major diagnostic groupings to meaningfully evaluate the relationship between symptoms and violence while taking diagnosis into account. To maximize the reliability and validity of the clinical diagnoses, data analysis used each patient's final discharge diagnosis, which had been reviewed by both the treating psychiatric resident and the supervising attending psychiatrist.

The Overt Aggression Scale (OAS) (17) was used to evaluate violent behavior exhibited by the patients in the hospital. The OAS is a widely used measure with documented reliability and validity as an index of inpatient aggression (18). It is a behavioral checklist that nursing staff complete at the end of each eight-hour shift to indicate if patients have engaged in physical aggression against other people, against objects, or against themselves or have engaged in verbal aggression. For our analysis, we limited the definition of violence to physical aggression against other people at some point during the patient's hospitalization.

The Brief Psychiatric Rating Scale (BPRS) (19), a widely used measure of psychopathology with good interrater reliability (20), was used to evaluate each patient at admission. Clinicians use the BPRS to rate patients on each of 18 symptom scales that range from 0, not present, to 6, extremely severe. In this study, ratings were made by psychiatric residents who had been trained in use of the BPRS and who were supervised closely by senior clinical staff. The senior clinical staff reviewed all BPRS forms to arrive at consensus ratings.

For purposes of data analysis, the BPRS symptom scales were combined into five summary scores described by Overall and Hollister (20). The summary scores are based on the following symptom clusters identified by factor analyses of the BPRS (20,21): thinking disturbance, which includes conceptual disorganization, hallucinatory behavior, and unusual thought content; anxious-depression, which includes guilt feelings, anxiety, and depressive mood; hostile-suspiciousness, which includes hostility, uncooperativeness, and suspiciousness; agitation-excitement, which includes tension and excitement; and withdrawal-retardation, which includes motor retardation, emotional withdrawal, and blunted affect.

To evaluate the relationship between symptoms observed at the time of admission and later violent behavior during hospitalization, scores on the five factor-based BPRS scales were compared for the assaultive and nonassaultive patients while diagnosis was taken into account. A two-way multivariate analysis of variance (MANOVA) was conducted; diagnosis and presence or absence of assaults were the independent variables, and the BPRS scores were the dependent variables. This approach minimizes the risk of inflation in the alpha level due to conducting multiple hypothesis tests. Statistical significance was assessed using Wilks' lambda, transformed into an F test.

Results

Characteristics

Fifty-four percent of the 330 patients were male. Seventy-one percent were Caucasian. The mean±SD age was 43.6±19 years, with a range from 15 to 95 years. Nineteen percent were married, 47 percent were single, and 34 percent were divorced, separated, or widowed. Seventy-three percent were in the lowest social class (Hollingshead's class V).

Primary diagnoses were based on *ICD-9-CM* criteria. Twenty-seven percent (N=89) had schizophrenic disorders, 18 percent (N=58) had manic disorders, 15 percent (N=49)

> *Twenty-three percent of the patients engaged in physical aggression against other people during their hospitalization. Assaultive patients were overrepresented in the diagnostic categories of schizophrenia, mania, and organic psychotic conditions.*

had organic psychotic conditions, and 41 percent (N=134) had other disorders. The other disorders included adjustment reactions (N=35), major depressive disorder (N=20), bipolar affective disorder, depressed (N=5), other nonorganic psychosis (N=12), unspecified psychosis (N=23), drug or alcohol dependence (N=13), neurotic disorders (N=11), personality disorders (N=6), and other disorders (N=9). Ninety-two percent of the patients were hospitalized on involuntary civil commitments.

Relationships between diagnosis, symptoms, and violence

Ratings on the OAS indicated that 23 percent of the patients (N=77) engaged in physical aggression against other people during their hospitalization. Assaultive patients were overrepresented in the diagnostic categories of schizophrenia, mania, and organic psychotic conditions (χ^2=18.52, df=3, p<.001). Thirty-six percent of the schizophrenic patients (N=32) became assaultive, as did 28 percent of the manic patients (N=16), 27 percent of patients with organic psychotic conditions (N=13), and 12 percent of patients with other disorders (N=16).

The two-way MANOVA showed significant main effects for violence and symptom patterns (F=7.81, df=5,318, p<.001), for diagnosis and symptoms (F=6.21, df=15,878, p<.001), and for the interaction between diagnosis and violence in relation to symptom patterns (F=1.70, df=15,878, p<.05). These results indicated that assaultive patients had significantly different symptom patterns than nonassaultive patients, that symptom patterns varied significantly across diagnostic groups, and that the symptom patterns associated with violence varied significantly across diagnostic groups.

Since the multivariate main effects were significant, we conducted separate two-way analyses of variance (ANOVAs) to examine the relationship of each symptom cluster to violence, diagnosis, and the interaction of violence and diagnosis. Compared with nonassaultive patients, patients who became assaultive had an admission mental status characterized by significantly higher levels of thinking disturbance (respective means were 7.44 and 8.75; F=5.10, df=1,322, p<.03), hostile-suspiciousness (respective means were 8.78 and 5.64; F=27.95, df=1,322, p<.001), and agitation-excitement (respective means were 5.56 and 4.17; F=11.14, df=1,322, p<.001). Assaultive and nonassaultive groups did not differ significantly on withdrawal-retardation (their respective means were 4.90 and 5.63) or anxious-depression (respective means were 6.19 and 6.72).

The interaction of diagnosis and violence in relation to symptom patterns was statistically significant for thinking disturbance (F=3.71, df=3,322, p<.02), hostile-suspiciousness (F=3.05, df=3,322, p<.03), and agitation-excitement (F=3.47, df=3, 322, p<.02). Table 1 illustrates the interaction of diagnosis and violence in relation to symptom patterns by showing the relationship between each symptom cluster and assaultive behavior, presented for each diagnostic group separately. Univariate analyses of variance (ANOVAs) of whether violent and nonviolent patients within a given diagnostic group differed on each symptom cluster are reported if the results of the analysis were significant. Even in cases where the univariate comparisons were not significant, the multivariate comparison indicated that the overall pattern of differences in the relation of assaultiveness to symptoms depending on diagnosis was significant for the thinking disturbance, hostile-suspiciousness, and agitation-excitement symptom clusters.

As shown in Table 1, higher levels of hostile-suspiciousness were associated with assaultiveness during hospitalization among patients with manic disorders, organic psychotic conditions, and other diagnoses, although this pattern was less pronounced among schizophrenic patients. Higher levels of agitation-excitement were associated with assaultiveness among patients with other diagnoses; however, this pattern was less marked for patients with organic psychotic conditions, schizophrenic patients, and manic patients. Higher levels of thinking disturbance were associated with assaultiveness among patients

Table 1

Mean Brief Psychiatric Rating Scale (BPRS) factor scores at admission for patients with various diagnoses who were assaultive or nonassaultive in the hospital[1]

Diagnosis	BPRS factor				
	Hostile-suspiciousness	Agitation-excitement	Thinking disturbance	Withdrawal-retardation	Anxious-depression
Schizophrenia					
Assaultive (N=32)	7.42	4.03	10.08	7.53	6.02
Nonassaultive (N=57)	6.81	3.91	10.42	6.51	6.27
Mania[2]					
Assaultive (N=16)	9.63	6.75	8.50	3.94	4.94
Nonassaultive (N=42)	6.38	5.67	8.36	3.19	5.83
Organic psychotic conditions[3]					
Assaultive (N=13)	8.38	4.38	7.85	3.97	5.92
Nonassaultive (N=36)	4.42	3.44	6.67	6.31	5.67
Other disorders[4]					
Assaultive (N=16)	9.69	7.06	8.56	4.75	7.88
Nonassaultive (N=118)	4.94	3.67	4.32	5.93	9.10

[1] Higher scores on the BPRS factors indicate higher levels of symptoms. Statistical comparisons assess differences between assaultive and nonassaultive patients within each diagnostic group, on each BPRS factor
[2] Significant difference between assaultive and nonassaultive manic patients in hostile-suspiciousness (F=5.61, df=1,56, p<.03)
[3] Significant difference between assaultive and nonassaultive patients with organic conditions in hostile-suspiciousness (F=8.20, df=1,47, p <.01)
[4] Significant differences between assaultive and nonassaultive patients with other mental disorders in hostile-suspiciousness (F=14.34, df=1,132, p<.001), agitation-excitement (F=21.20, df=1,132, p<.001), and thinking disturbance (F=14.34, df=1,132, p<.001)

with other diagnoses, whereas this pattern was less marked for patients with manic disorders or organic psychotic conditions and was absent for schizophrenic patients. Neither a main effect for assaultiveness nor an interaction of assaultiveness and diagnosis was present for withdrawal-retardation or anxious-depression.

As a check on the validity of the diagnostic groupings, the main effect for diagnosis on each BPRS symptom scale was also examined. As expected, the diagnostic groups differed significantly in levels of thinking disturbance ($F=10.56$, $df=3,322$, $p<.001$), withdrawal-retardation ($F=7.58$, $df=3,322$, $p<.001$), anxious-depression ($F=7.31$, $df=3,322$, $p<.001$), and agitation-excitement ($F=7.39$, $df=3,322$, $p<.001$).

Post hoc comparisons using Bonferroni t tests showed several significant differences ($p<.05$) between diagnostic groups. Schizophrenic patients had significantly higher levels of thinking disturbance than the three other diagnostic groups, and higher levels of withdrawal-retardation than patients with manic disorders and organic psychotic conditions. Manic patients had higher levels of agitation-excitement than the three other diagnostic groups, and lower levels of withdrawal-retardation than patients with schizophrenia or other diagnoses. Patients with other diagnoses had higher levels of anxious-depression and lower levels of thinking disturbance, compared with patients with schizophrenia, mania, or organic psychotic conditions. Overall, these symptom patterns are compatible with symptom patterns that would be expected based on *ICD-9-CM* and *DSM-III-R* criteria for these diagnostic groups.

Discussion and conclusions

Consistent with previous research (7–9,22), this study found an association between diagnoses such as schizophrenia, mania, and organic psychotic conditions and imminent risk of assaultive behavior among a sample of acutely ill, newly hospitalized patients. Similarly, increased risk of violence was associated with higher levels of hostile-suspiciousness, thinking disturbance, and agitation-excitement. However, the value of these symptom clusters as indicators of imminent violence varied with the patient's diagnosis.

For example, the level of hostile-suspiciousness at admission was much higher among assaultive patients with manic disorders, organic psychotic conditions, and other mental disorders than among nonassaultive patients with those disorders. However, among patients with schizophrenia, there were no significant differences in the level of hostile-suspiciousness between patients who later became assaultive and those who did not. It is noteworthy that several previous studies with samples comprised primarily of schizophrenic patients have failed to identify an association between hostility and violence (23–25) and have hypothesized that hostility is of little utility as an indicator of risk of violence in acute treatment settings.

By taking into account appropriate control groups, our findings suggest that for most acute patients the level of hostile-suspiciousness is generally a useful indicator of imminent risk of violence. However, hostility may be a less useful indicator of the potential for violence among schizophrenic patients. This difference could be due to staff's more active treatment of hostile and paranoid schizophrenic patients or to increased responsiveness of schizophrenic patients to the pharmacological and psychosocial components of hospital treatment.

The superiority of clinical variables in predicting violence in the hospital might be explained by the fact that an increase in symptoms is typically considered in the decision to admit patients to the hospital.

These findings suggest that symptom profiles represent a useful level of analysis for understanding the relationship between violence and psychopathology. Because the severity of many mental disorders, such as manic and schizophrenic disorders, fluctuates over time, psychopathological variables may be most pertinent to assessing risk of violence when the patient is symptomatic. This possibility could explain the limited usefulness that diagnosis has had in predicting violence among outpatients, since patients are less likely to be severely symptomatic in outpatient settings. In fact, when symptoms have been directly assessed in outpatient samples, symptom profiles have been more powerful than demographic characteristics as predictors of violence (26,27).

Similarly, clinical variables have proved superior to demographic variables in identifying short-term risk of violence among hospitalized patients (6). The superiority of clinical variables in predicting violence in the hospital might be explained by the fact that an increase in symptoms is typically considered in the decision to admit patients to the hospital (28,29).

The issue is complicated by the fact that some diagnostic categories, such as schizophrenia, are characterized by high levels of symptoms, such as thinking disturbance, that are generally related to increased risk of violence. On the one hand, this association could account for the higher proportion of assaultive patients among patients with schizophrenia. On the other hand, to the extent that clinical staff accurately identify schizophrenic patients with high levels of symptoms such as thinking disturbance, treatment interventions may be initiated to target the symptoms and thereby reduce their utility as markers of risk of violence within that diagnostic group. Such a formulation could explain why thinking disturbance did not differentiate violent from nonviolent schizophrenic patients, despite being generally related to risk of violence in the sample as a whole.

Additional research is needed to

identify markers for risk of assaultiveness among schizophrenic patients for whom treatment interventions have already targeted obvious indicators of aggressiveness such as hostility, uncooperativeness, and suspiciousness. Such research might also include assessment of aspects of staff-patient interactions or other features of the treatment milieu that influence the expression of assaultive behavior (30).

The inconsistent findings of previous studies examining the relationship between mental disorder and violence may partly reflect research designs that failed to include appropriate control groups. To our knowledge, our study is the first to include control groups with different diagnoses in an evaluation of relationships between acute symptomatology and violence. The study findings suggest the value of specific symptom profiles in identifying patients at risk for violence.

Our study design represents a refinement over past research on psychopathology and violence, which has typically evaluated diagnosis without reference to changes in mental status (31) or changes in mental status without regard to diagnosis (32). Further research is needed to examine the implications of treatments received by patients with different diagnoses for amelioration of specific symptoms that are associated with risk of assault. ♦

Acknowledgment

This work was partly supported by grant S07-RR05755 from the biomedical research support grant program of the Division of Research Resources at the National Institutes of Health.

References

1. Monahan J: Risk assessment of violence among the mentally disordered: generating useful knowledge. International Journal of Law and Psychiatry 11:249–257, 1988
2. Otto R: The prediction of dangerous behavior: a review and analysis of "second-generation" research. Forensic Reports 5:103–133, 1992
3. McNiel DE, Binder RL: Clinical assessment of the risk of violence among psychiatric inpatients. American Journal of Psychiatry 148:1317–1321, 1991
4. Swanson JW, Holzer CE, Ganju VK, et al: Violence and psychiatric disorder in the community: evidence from the Epidemiologic Catchment Area surveys. Hospital and Community Psychiatry 41:761–770, 1990
5. McNiel DE, Binder RL, Greenfield TK: Predictors of violence in civilly committed acute psychiatric patients. American Journal of Psychiatry 145:965–978, 1988
6. Rossi AM, Jacobs M, Monteleone M, et al: Characteristics of patients who engage in assaultive or other fear-inducing behavior. Journal of Nervous and Mental Disease 174:154–160, 1986
7. Krakowski M, Volavka J, Brizer D: Psychopathology and violence: a review of the literature. Comprehensive Psychiatry 27:131–148, 1986
8. Kalunian DA, Binder RL, McNiel DE: Violence in geriatric patients who need psychiatric hospitalization. Journal of Clinical Psychiatry 51:340–343, 1990
9. Binder RL, McNiel DE: Effects of diagnosis and context on dangerousness. American Journal of Psychiatry 145:728–732, 1988
10. Monahan J: Mental disorder and violent behavior: perceptions and evidence. American Psychologist 47:511–521, 1992
11. McNiel DE: Violence and hallucinations, in Violence and Mental Disorder: Developments in Risk Assessment. Edited by Monahan J, Steadman H. Chicago, University of Chicago Press, in press
12. Tanke ED, Yesavage JA: Characteristics of assaultive patients who do and do not provide cues to potential violence. American Journal of Psychiatry 142:1409–1413, 1985
13. Yesavage JA: Inpatient violence and the schizophrenic patient. Acta Psychiatrica Scandinavica 67:353–357, 1983
14. Yesavage J: Bipolar illness: correlates of dangerous inpatient behavior. British Journal of Psychiatry 143:554–557, 1983
15. Lion JR, Snyder W, Merrill GL: Underreporting of assaults on staff in a state hospital. Hospital and Community Psychiatry 32:497–498, 1981
16. Lowenstein M, Binder RL, McNiel DE: The relationship between admission symptoms and hospital assaults. Hospital and Community Psychiatry 41:311–313, 1990
17. Yudofsky SC, Silver JM, Jackson W, et al: The Overt Aggression Scale for the objective rating of verbal and physical aggression. American Journal of Psychiatry 143:35–39, 1986
18. Silver JM, Yudofsky SC: The Overt Aggression Scale: overview and guiding principles. Journal of Neuropsychiatry and Clinical Neurosciences 3:S22–S29, 1991
19. Overall J, Gorham DR: The Brief Psychiatric Rating Scale. Psychological Reports 10:799–812, 1962
20. Overall JE, Hollister JE: Assessment of depression using the Brief Psychiatric Rating Scale, in Assessment of Depression. Edited by Satorius N, Ban TA. New York, Springer-Verlag, 1986
21. Hedlund JL, Vieweg MS: The Brief Psychiatric Rating Scale: a comprehensive review. Journal of Operational Psychiatry 11:48–65, 1980
22. Beck JC, Bonnar J: Emergency civil commitment: predicting hospital violence from behavior in the community. Journal of Psychiatry and the Law 16:379–388, 1988
23. Yesavage JA, Werner PD, Becker JMT, et al: Short-term civil commitment and the violent patient. American Journal of Psychiatry 139:1145–1149, 1982
24. Werner PD, Rose TL, Yesavage JA: Reliability, accuracy, and decision-making strategy in clinical predictions of imminent dangerousness. Journal of Consulting and Clinical Psychology 51:815–825, 1983
25. Krakowski M, Jaeger J, Volavka J: Violence and psychopathology: a longitudinal study. Comprehensive Psychiatry 29:174–181, 1986
26. Link BG, Andrews H, Cullen FT: The violent and illegal behavior of mental patients reconsidered. American Sociological Review 57:275–292, 1992
27. Bartels SJ, Drake RE, Wallach MA, et al: Characteristic hostility in schizophrenic outpatients. Schizophrenia Bulletin 17:163–171, 1991
28. McNiel DE, Myers R, Zeiner H, et al: The role of violence in decisions about hospitalization from the psychiatric emergency room. American Journal of Psychiatry 149:207–212, 1992
29. Beck JC, White KA, Gage B: Emergency psychiatric assessment of violence. American Journal of Psychiatry 148:1562–1565, 1991
30. Binder RL, McNiel DE: Staff gender and risk of assault on doctors and nurses. Presented at the annual meeting of the American Academy of Psychiatry and the Law, San Antonio, Texas, Oct 21–24, 1993
31. Tardiff K, Sweillam A: Assault, suicide, and mental illness. Archives of General Psychiatry 37:164–169, 1980
32. Palmstierna T, Lassenius R, Wistedt B: Evaluation of the Brief Psychopathological Rating Scale in relation to aggressive behavior by acute involuntarily admitted patients. Acta Psychiatrica Scandinavica 79:313–316, 1989

A Prospective Study of Violence by Psychiatric Patients After Hospital Discharge

Kenneth Tardiff, M.D., M.P.H.
Peter M. Marzuk, M.D.
Andrew C. Leon, Ph.D.
Laura Portera, B.A.

The public fears violence by patients who are discharged from psychiatric hospitals. This fear has been fueled by newspaper accounts of released psychiatric patients stabbing strangers on the street or pushing helpless victims from train platforms. Both clinicians and hospital administrators are aware of the legal liability in premature or inappropriate hospital discharge and the need to protect potential victims from violence by their patients (1–4). Clinicians should be knowledgeable about risk factors for violence by psychiatric patients after discharge to make appropriate decisions about the timing of discharge and to plan aftercare services in the community.

Surprisingly few studies have examined violence by psychiatric patients immediately after discharge from the hospital. Some studies have done a follow-up of special populations such as those who had undergone court-ordered psychiatric assessments after criminal behavior (5–7) or violent offenders who had been released from prison or forensic hospitals (8,9). Others have studied men admitted to psychiatric hospitals who were judged to be potentially violent before discharge (10–12). Studies of more general, heterogeneous patient populations are limited. A pilot study from a collaborative group assessed the frequency of violence by patients released from psychiatric hospitals, but the risk factors analyzed so far are only demographic and not clinical ones (13). One study followed patients for six months after they were seen in an emergency department and assessed the risk of violence toward other persons (14).

These prospective studies have followed patients for months or years after discharge rather than focusing on a

Objective: The study assessed the frequency of violence by patients two weeks after discharge from a psychiatric hospital and identified characteristics of patients with an increased risk of violence after discharge. *Methods:* A structured form was used to interview patients aged 18 to 59 years in a private university psychiatric hospital. Patients provided self-reports of past violence, and violence while in the hospital was assessed by routine nurse ratings. Patients were telephoned two weeks after discharge to assess violence since discharge. *Results:* Sixteen of 430 patients who were interviewed by telephone two weeks after discharge reported violence against persons since their discharge. Patients who were violent in the month before admission were nine times more likely to be violent in the two weeks after discharge, compared with patients who were not violent just before admission. Patients with a personality disorder were four times more likely than patients without a personality disorder to be violent after discharge. The targets of violence were often family members or other intimates and often the same persons attacked before hospitalization. *Conclusions:* Patients who were violent just before admission were more likely to be violent after discharge and to attack the same persons they had attacked in the past. Clinicians should routinely evaluate past violence and work with the patient and potential targets of violence to prevent future violence.

When this paper was published the authors were affiliated with the department of psychiatry at Cornell University Medical College in New York City. From the May 1997 issue of Psychiatric Services *(volume 48, pages 678–681).*

shorter term, such as one or two weeks, which is of greater clinical and legal relevance in decision-making. Short-term prediction of risk is important when a clinician must decide whether a patient can be sent home from the emergency room and when an outpatient's potential for violence is monitored from office visit to office visit.

The study reported here has focused on the short-term assessment of the risk of violence in a general heterogenous population of psychiatric patients discharged from a psychiatric hospital. We assessed the frequency and types of violence by discharged patients and assessed the characteristics of patients who were violent after discharge from the hospital.

Methods

All patients between 18 and 59 years of age who were admitted consecutively to the Payne Whitney Clinic, a private university psychiatric hospital in Manhattan, during an 18-month period were eligible for the study. Of the 1,068 patients admitted during the study period, 102 refused to give informed consent, and 203 could not be interviewed due to their illness or because they were discharged before an interview could take place. Thus the study group consisted of 763 subjects.

A trained research assistant gave a complete description of the study to the subjects and obtained their written informed consent to participate. A comparison of participants and nonparticipants revealed no significant differences in age, gender, race, psychiatric diagnosis, or socioeconomic status.

A trained research assistant administered a closed-ended structured interview instrument that included questions about demographic and socioeconomic characteristics and any history of violence and alcohol and drug use. (A copy of the assessment form is available from the authors.) Demographic data obtained from the patient were subsequently verified using the patient's chart.

The senior author determined axis I and II diagnoses for all patients at discharge, using information from patients' charts and *DSM-III-R* criteria.

Of the 16 patients who were violent after discharge, 13 had been violent one or more times in the past.

Patients were grouped into categories by diagnosis. The majority of patients in the schizophrenia category had a diagnosis of schizophrenia; some had brief reactive psychosis, atypical psychosis, or delusional disorder. In the category of mania, most patients had a diagnosis of bipolar disorder, manic, and a few had cyclothymia. The depression category included predominantly patients with major depression and a few with dysthymia. Roughly half of the patients in the category of other axis I disorders were diagnosed with adjustment disorder.

Violence toward persons in the month preceding admission was assessed by asking the patient whether he or she was physically violent toward persons or objects and, if so, what was the target, the means of inflicting injury, the severity of injury to the target, and the circumstances of the violent encounter. Nurses rated patients' behavior each day while they were in the hospital, and the ratings were included in the computerized inpatient record. One item on the rating instrument assessed if the patient was physically violent toward other persons.

Two weeks after discharge the patients were telephoned by the research assistant. During the telephone interview, the patient was asked about any violent acts during the two weeks after discharge from the hospital. The same form used to assesss violence in the month before admission was used to record violence after discharge. Information was gathered about postdischarge compliance with prescribed medication and the use of alcohol and illicit drugs.

Two-tailed chi square tests were used to compare the characteristics of patients who were interviewed and not interviewed and to compare patients who were violent in the two weeks after discharge with those who were not violent during that period. The level set for significance was <.05.

Results

Of the 763 patients participating in the study, 430, or 56.3 percent, were interviewed after discharge. Patients who were not interviewed were more likely to be nonwhite than were the interviewees (47.4 percent versus 36.6 percent, $\chi^2=10.70$, df=3, p=.01). Patients who were interviewed were slightly more likely to have a history of violence in the month before admission to the hospital (51.9 percent versus 48.1 percent, $\chi^2=3.91$, df=1, p=.05). No significant differences in age, gender, diagnosis, presence of violence while in the hospital, or history of violent ideation were found between patients who were interviewed after discharge and those who were not interviewed.

Among the 430 patients who were interviewed, 16 (3.7 percent) reported one or more violent acts toward persons within two weeks after discharge. Most of the attacks were directed toward spouses, other intimates, or other family members. Most of the attacks involved punching or scratching and left minor bruises or scratches. One patient tried to strangle his spouse. Four attacks targeted people who were not patients' relatives or intimates. They involved an armed robbery, pushing a stranger on the street, punching a roommate, and scratching and pulling the hair of a stranger during an argument in a store.

The characteristics of the patients who were violent and nonviolent after discharge are presented in Table 1. Patients with an axis II disorder were more likely to be violent after discharge, compared with those with no axis II disorder. Patients with borderline or antisocial personality disorders were four times more likely, and patients with other types of personality disorders were 2.3 times more likely, to be violent than patients without a personality disorder. Patients who were violent toward persons in the month before admission were 9.1 times more likely to be violent toward persons after discharge.

There were no statistically significant differences between violent and nonviolent patients in gender, race, or the presence of schizophrenia, mania, depression, substance abuse, other organic disorders, or other axis I disorders. The two groups also did not differ in self-reported compliance with medication or in the use of alcohol or drugs after discharge. Having been violent in the hospital did not differentiate patients who were violent from those who were not violent after discharge. In fact, none of the patients who were physically violent during hospitalization were violent after discharge.

Of the 16 patients who were violent after discharge, 13 (81.3 percent) had a history of one or more violent episodes some time in the past. Half of those incidents occurred more than one month before admission. For nine of those patients (69.2 percent), the target of past violence was the same person—most often a spouse, other intimate, or other family member—who was attacked by the patient after hospital discharge.

Discussion

A small but alarming number of the patients in our study, 3.7 percent, were violent within two weeks after hospital discharge. Unlike incidents of violence involving psychiatric patients that are reported in the media, attacks by patients in this study were not likely to target strangers in public places. Rather, spouses, other intimates, and other family members were the typical targets.

Our study found a lower percentage of patients with self-reported violence after discharge than have other studies (12–14). This difference is probably partly due to the much longer follow-up periods in those studies. In addition, our study probably underreports violence after discharge because of the disproportionate number of patients with a history of violence before admission who were not able to be contacted after discharge and because we relied on self-reports of violence. As has been shown in other studies (5,9,10), we found that patients with a history of violence before admission were more likely to be violent after discharge.

Type of axis I disorder was not related to risk of violence after discharge. Most likely, axis I pathology had been treated during the hospital stay and symptoms would not be expected to reappear immediately after discharge. In earlier studies, axis I pathology was found to be associated with violence just before admission, probably due to noncompliance with medication and emergence of psychosis or mania (15–19).

In contrast, patients with personality disorders were four times more likely than those without personality disorders to be violent after discharge. Pathology associated with personality disorders is generally not amenable to medication and can be considered trait rather than state phenomena. For the patients in our study, axis II pathology appeared to persist after discharge and to be manifested in interpersonal conflict, particularly with persons close to the patient, and in low frustration tolerance, an exaggerated sense of entitlement, and difficulties in the patient's verbal expression of emotional turmoil.

Table 1

Characteristics of psychiatric patients who were violent and were not violent toward persons after hospital discharge

Characteristic	Violent (N=16)		Not violent (N=414)	
	N	%	N	%
Age (years)				
18 to 29	8	6.0	125	94.0
30 to 39	5	3.4	142	96.6
40 to 49	2	2.2	89	97.8
50 to 59	1	1.7	58	98.3
Gender				
Male	4	2.0	192	98.0
Female	12	5.1	222	94.9
Race				
White	9	3.3	265	96.7
African American	4	5.6	68	94.4
Latino	2	3.0	65	97.0
Asian and other	1	5.9	16	94.1
Schizophrenia				
Present	2	2.2	90	97.8
Absent	14	4.1	324	95.9
Mania				
Present	3	4.2	68	95.8
Absent	13	3.6	346	96.4
Depression				
Present	5	2.9	168	97.1
Absent	11	4.3	246	95.7
Substance abuse				
Present	4	4.5	84	95.5
Absent	12	3.5	330	96.5
Other organic disorder				
Present	0	0	21	100.0
Absent	16	3.9	393	96.1
Other axis I disorder				
Present	3	4.6	62	95.4
Absent	13	3.6	352	96.4
Axis II disorder[1]				
Borderline or antisocial personality disorder	4	9.5	38	90.5
Other axis II disorder	5	5.6	85	94.4
No axis II disorder	7	2.4	290	97.6
Violence toward persons within the month before admission[2]				
Present	9	17.3	43	82.7
Absent	7	1.9	371	98.1

[1] Significant difference between groups, $\chi^2=6.32$, df=2, p=.04
[2] Significant difference between groups, $\chi^2=30.48$, df=1, p<.001

Violence by the patient in the hospital was not related to later violence after discharge. Violence in the hospital was probably due to the state of the patient as a result of axis I pathology or to specific circumstances or environmental factors unique to the hospital. Thus past violence in the hospital should not delay discharge as long as the patient is stable and no longer considered a risk for violence.

In our study, persons attacked by patients after discharge had usually been attacked before the patient was hospitalized. This finding underscores the need to evaluate past violence by patients. The clinician should routinely ask the patient about ideas of violence and actual episodes of violence. Questions such as "Have you ever lost your temper?" and "Have you ever thought about violence toward others?" should be as routine in a clinical interview as "Have you ever attempted suicide?" and "Have you ever thought of killing yourself?"

If the patient has thought of being violent, a complete assessment of violence ideation should be made, much the same way as suicidal ideation is assessed. The clinician should assess the patient's degree of planning, available means, and access to the potential victim. If violence has occurred more than once, the clinician should attempt to delineate similarities in these incidents to develop strategies to prevent future violence.

While the patient in is the hospital, the clinician should work with the patient and persons who have been attacked to develop strategies for prevention. Ideally, this work could be done in sessions involving both the perpetrator and victim of violence, so past patterns of violence could be reviewed. Other family members or significant others who played a role in past violent confrontations could be involved in these sessions. Useful techniques of evaluation and psychotherapy for violent patients are discussed in greater detail elsewhere (20).

Conclusions

Violence by psychiatric patients shortly after hospital discharge was increased among patients with personality disorders and those who had a history of violence toward persons before being admitted to the hospital. Often the target of violence after discharge was the same person, often an intimate or family member, who was attacked by the patient before hospitalization. Clinicians should routinely evaluate past violence and work with the patient and family to prevent future violence after discharge. ◆

Acknowledgments

This work was partly supported by the Aaron Diamond Foundation and the DeWitt-Wallace New York Community Fund.

References

1. Poythress NG: Avoiding negligent release: contemporary clinical and risk management strategies. American Journal of Psychiatry 147:994–997, 1990
2. Appelbaum PS: Tarasoff and the clinician: problems in fulfilling the duty to protect. American Journal of Psychiatry 142:425–429, 1985
3. Beck JC: The Potentially Violent Patient and the Tarasoff Decision. Washington, DC, American Psychiatric Press, 1985
4. Mills MJ, Sullivan G, Eth S: Protecting third parties: a decade after Tarasoff. American Journal of Psychiatry 144:68–74, 1987
5. Sepejak D, Menzies RJ, Webster CD, et al: Clinical predictions of dangerousness: a two-year follow-up of 408 pre-trial forensic cases. Bulletin of the American Academy of Psychiatry and Law 11:171–181, 1983
6. Webster CD, Sepejak DS, Menzies RJ, et al: The reliability and validity of dangerousness predictions. Bulletin of the American Academy of Psychiatry and Law 12:41–50, 1984
7. Menzies RJ, Webster CD, Sepejak DS: The dimensions of dangerousness: evaluating the accuracy of psychometric predictions of violence among forensic patients. Law and Human Behavior 9:49–70, 1985
8. Eronen M, Hokola P, Tiihonen J: Factors associated with homicide recidivism in a 13-year sample of homicide offenders in Finland. Psychiatric Services 47:403–406, 1996
9. De Jong J, Virkkunen M, Linnoila M: Factors associated with recidivism in a criminal population. Journal of Nervous and Mental Disease 180:543–550, 1992
10. Klassen D, O'Conner WA: A prospective study of predictors of violence in adult mental health admissions. Law and Human Behavior 12:143–158, 1988
11. Klassen D, O'Conner WA: Crime, inpatient admissions, and violence among male patients. International Journal of Law and Psychiatry 11:305–312, 1988
12. Klassen D, O'Conner WA: Assessing risk of violence in released mental patients: a cross-validation study. Psychological Assessment 1:75–81, 1989
13. Steadman HJ, Monahan J, Appelbaum PS, et al: Designing a new generation of risk assessment research, in Violence and Mental Disorder: Developments in Risk Assessment. Edited by Monahan J, Steadman HJ. Chicago, University of Chicago Press, 1994
14. Lidz CW, Mulvey EP, Gardner W: The accuracy of predictions of violence to others. JAMA 269:1007–1011, 1993
15. Tardiff K, Sweillam A: Assault, suicide, and mental illness. Archives of General Psychiatry 37:164–169, 1980
16. Craig TJ: An epidemiologic study of problems associated with violence among psychiatric patients. American Journal of Psychiatry 139:1262–1266, 1982
17. Taylor PJ, Gunn J: Violence and psychosis: I. risk of violence among psychotic men. British Medical Journal 288:1945–1949, 1984
18. Rossi AM, Jacobs M, Monteleone M, et al: Violent or fear-inducing behavior associated with hospital admission. Hospital and Community Psychiatry 36:643–647, 1985
19. Binder RL, McNeil DE: Effects of diagnosis and context on dangerousness. American Journal of Psychiatry 145:728–732, 1988
20. Tardiff K: Assessment and Management of Violent Patients, 2nd ed. Washington, DC, American Psychiatric Press, 1996

Early-Onset Substance Abuse and Community Violence by Outpatients With Chronic Mental Illness

Carl Fulwiler, M.D., Ph.D.
Hillel Grossman, M.D.
Catherine Forbes, B.A.
Robin Ruthazer, M.P.H.

Recent studies have consistently found that violence is more common among people with mental illness compared with the general population (1–3). This finding contrasts with earlier studies, illustrated in Rabkin's review (4) of the older literature. Although the violence attributed to mentally ill persons accounts for only a small fraction of the violence in our society (5), it is a major reason for psychiatric hospitalization and involuntary commitment (6,7).

The Epidemiologic Catchment Area (ECA) study used structured interviews to survey the prevalence of psychiatric illness in a large, unselected sample of the United States population (8). A separate analysis of the survey responses pertaining to violent behavior revealed that the lifetime prevalence of violence among people with either schizophrenia or major affective disorder was almost double the rate among people without these conditions (1).

In a large, unselected birth cohort in Sweden, Hodgins (3) examined national registries to identify those who developed mental illness and those registered as committing crimes by age 30. Of the subjects with major mental illness, 14.6 percent had been arrested for a violent crime, compared with 5.7 percent of subjects without major mental illness. Lindqvist and Allebeck (9) did a 15-year follow-up study of a population-based cohort of all inpatients with a diagnosis of schizophrenia who were discharged from hospitals in Stockholm in 1971 (N=664). They used criminal registries to determine the number of arrests. The incidence of violent crimes was four times higher than in the general population.

The increased risk for violence among persons with mental illness remains significant when demographic factors and socioeconomic status are taken into account (1,3). The reasons for the increased risk of violence associated with mental illness are not

Objective: This study examined the relationship between violence and substance abuse among patients with chronic mental illness living in the community. *Methods:* All referrals over a one-year period to an urban assertive community treatment team were evaluated systematically with a standardized intake protocol. Thirty-seven patients with a history of violence in the community were compared with 27 patients without such a history on a variety of clinical and demographic variables. *Results:* More than half of the patients (58 percent) had a history of violence in the community. The only significant differences between those with a history of violence and those without involved alcohol or drug use. The single best predictor of violence was the onset of alcohol or drug abuse in late childhood or early adolescence. *Conclusions:* In this sample, very early onset of substance abuse among people who developed mental illness was associated with the greatest risk of community violence. Thus at least some of the causal determinants of violence in this sample may precede the onset of adult mental illness.

Dr. Fulwiler, Dr. Grossman, and *Ms. Forbes* are affiliated with the department of psychiatry at Tufts University School of Medicine and New England Medical Center in Boston. *Ms. Ruthazer* is with the division of clinical care research of the Tufts University School of Medicine in Boston. From the September 1997 issue of Psychiatric Services (volume 48, pages 1181–1185).

Table 1

Demographic and clinical characteristics of violent and nonviolent patients with chronic mental illness

Characteristic	Violent (N=37)	Nonviolent (N=27)	Value	df	p[1]
Age (mean±SD years)	37.16±7.79	46.33±12.77	t=3.56	62	.001
Education (mean±SD years)	9.77±2.32	10.41±2.72	t=.98	59	ns
Age at first psychiatric diagnosis (mean±SD years)	20.21±6.30	31.73±16.19	t=3.70	56	.000
Duration of illness (mean±SD years)	16.65±9.68	14.00±9.67	t=−1.05	58	ns
Male (%)	86.5	51.9	χ^2=9.2	1	.002
Homeless at intake (%)	70.3	40.7	χ^2=5.58	1	.018
History of a suicide attempt (%)[2]	57.1	22.2	χ^2=7.63	1	.006

[1] Raw p values. Applying the Bonferroni correction for possible type I error, a raw p value of <.001 is significant at p<.05 level.
[2] Data not available for two subjects

known. A major risk factor is substance abuse. In the ECA study, substance abuse almost doubled the lifetime prevalence of violence among persons with mental illness (1). In the Swedish birth cohort, alcohol or drug abuse was present among 48.7 percent of the violent group of mentally ill persons (3). In the long-term follow-up of patients with schizophrenia in Sweden, 55 percent of the patients registered for violence during the follow-up period had definite or probable alcohol abuse (10).

These findings have led some researchers to conclude that the increased rate of violence among mentally ill persons can largely be attributed to the subgroup with comorbid substance abuse disorders (11). However, whether substances make people with mental illness more violent or whether both substance abuse and violence are increased in a particular subgroup of mentally ill persons is unknown.

The purpose of the study reported here was to further explore the relationship between substance abuse and violence among people with chronic mental illness in an effort to identify clinical or demographic factors that might define a more homogeneous subgroup with the highest risk.

Methods

Subjects for this study were all referrals over a one-year period (September 1, 1994, to August 31, 1995) to the Baycove–New England Medical Center community treatment team. The community treatment team serves the Baycove Mental Health Center catchment area in Boston, comprising primarily low-income inner-city neighborhoods. The community treatment team is contracted by the state to provide intensive community-based mental health services, following the model of the Program for Assertive Community Treatment developed in Madison, Wisconsin (12,13).

Referrals are made by state mental health agencies. To be eligible for the program, patients must have severe mental illness and must have required multiple hospitalizations during the previous two years. A total of 90 patients were referred to the program during the study period. Twenty-six either were never located or had to be exluded for lack of sufficient information because they refused to be interviewed and records were not available. The final sample consisted of 64 patients.

Clinical and demographic data were collected using a standardized intake protocol administered by one of the two psychiatrists on the research team (CF or HG). The protocol included a semistructured interview, an interview of a family member when possible, and a review of all available hospital and outpatient records. Arrest records were available for 12 subjects. Diagnoses were made by the interviewing psychiatrist using *DSM-IV* criteria (14).

For this study, violence was defined as committing physical or sexual battery against another person in the community, excluding acts of self-defense. Only incidents that occurred after age 18 and after the patient had received a psychiatric diagnosis, or that led directly to the first psychiatric diagnosis, were counted. Inpatient assaults were excluded because staff practices have been shown to influence the incidence (15) and reporting (16) of such events. The sources for this information on violence included self-report, a careful review of all available psychiatric records, and, when possible, a review of criminal records. Threats of violence or assault without physical contact were not counted.

Patients with a history of violence were compared with the remaining patients on clinical and demographic variables. Continuous variables were analyzed using t tests, and chi square tests were performed on dichotomous variables. The results are presented as raw p values. Possible type I error is also discussed in terms of a conservative Bonferroni correction for the number of variables examined (a total of 50 variables), considering a corrected p value of <.05 as significant. Logistic regression was used to examine multivariate relationships among variables pertaining to mental illness and substance abuse. The software used for statistical analysis was SAS, version 6.12 for Windows.

Results

The mean±SD age of the sample was 41±11 years. Seventy-one percent were male, and 58 percent were homeless. Forty-six percent were Caucasian, and 43 percent were African American. The mean±SD number of years of education was 10±2.5.

Psychiatric diagnoses were schizophrenia, for 36 percent; bipolar I disorder, for 19 percent; schizoaffective disorder, for 11 percent; substance abuse, for 11 percent; severe personality disorder, for 6 percent; adult attention deficit disorder and bipolar II disorder, each for 3 percent; and dementia, major depression with psychotic features, obsessive-compulsive disorder, and mood disorder due to a general medical condition, each for

Table 2

DSM-IV psychiatric diagnoses of violent and nonviolent patients with and without a history of substance abuse

| | Violent (N=37) | | | Nonviolent (N=27) | | |
| | | Substance abuse | | | Substance abuse | |
Diagnosis	Total	Yes	No	Total	Yes	No
Schizophrenia	11	10	1	12	2	10
Bipolar I disorder	6	6	0	6	4	2
Schizoaffective disorder	6	6	0	1	0	1
Substance dependence	6	—	—	1	—	—
Alcohol dependence	2	—	—	1	—	—
Attention-deficit/hyperactivity (adult)	2	2	0	0	—	—
Dementia	1	1	0	0	—	—
Major depressive disorder	1	1	0	0	—	—
Bipolar II disorder	0	—	—	2	2	0
Obsessive-compulsive disorder	0	—	—	1	0	1
Personality disorder not otherwise specified	0	—	—	1	0	1
Mood disorder due to medical condition	0	—	—	1	0	1
Borderline personality	2	1	1	1	0	1

1.5 percent. Seventy-seven percent of the sample had a history of an alcohol or drug use disorder. Patients who fulfilled criteria for both a mental illness and a substance use disorder were considered to have dual diagnoses. For 16 percent of the referrals, a mood or psychotic disorder was considered to be substance induced.

A history of interpersonal violence in the community after the onset of adult mental illness was common in the sample (58 percent), and the most common victims were nonrelatives. The most frequent act of violence was simple battery. Twenty-two percent of patients used a weapon, and 8 percent committed rape or attempted rape. One patient had been charged with attempted murder. All violent subjects had more than one documented instance of violence as defined; most had three or more incidents.

As Table 1 shows, violent patients were more likely to be male, to have a history of a suicide attempt, and to be homeless and younger at the time of referral. They were also younger when their mental illness was first diagnosed, but the length of illness was the same as for nonviolent patients. Making a conservative correction for type I error, only age at first diagnosis remained significant (corrected p value $<.05$).

Table 2 shows the *DSM-IV* diagnoses of violent and nonviolent patients. No significant differences were found in the rate of violence within diagnostic groups. However, a history of a comorbid substance use disorder—substance abuse or dependence—appeared to be strongly associated with an increased risk of violence.

The contribution of substance disorders to the risk of violence in people with mental illness was further explored by grouping psychiatric disorders into two categories—major mental illness, consisting of schizophrenia, schizoaffective disorder, bipolar disorder, and major depressive disorder; and other diagnoses. Overall, patients with major mental illness were not significantly more likely to be violent than patients with other diagnoses (52 percent versus 56 percent). Major mental illness alone, with no history of alcohol or drug abuse, was associated with a significantly lower risk of violence (Table 3). Only 7 percent of patients with major mental illness alone had a history of violence, compared with 73 percent of patients who had both a major mental illness and a history of substance abuse. The effect of a history of substance abuse was similar for patients with major mental illness and those with other disorders. Thus in this sample mental illness was not associated with violence unless it was accompanied by a history of substance abuse.

As for the contribution of major mental illness to the risk of violence associated with substance abuse, the rate of violence was similar whether major mental illness was present or not (Table 3). To examine this relationship further, we performed a logistic regression that included the factors major mental illness and substance abuse and the interaction between them. We found no evidence of

Table 3

Major mental illness and alcohol and drug abuse among violent and nonviolent patients

| | Violent (N=37) | | Nonviolent (N=27) | | | |
Variable	N	%	N	%	χ^2	p[1]
Any major mental illness	25	52	23	48	2.58	ns
Major mental illness with alcohol or drug abuse	24	73	9	27	6.21	.01
Major mental illness without alcohol or drug abuse	1	7	14	93	21.01	$<.001$
Any alcohol or drug abuse	35	75	12	25	20.13	$<.001$
Alcohol or drug abuse without major mental illness	6	86	1	14	2.51	ns
Onset of alcohol or drug abuse before age 15[2]	21	91	2	9	18.93	$<.001$

[1] Raw p values; df=1 for all comparisons. Applying the Bonferroni correction for possible type I error, a raw p value of $<.001$ is significant at $p<.05$ level.
[2] Data not available for four subjects

an interaction between major mental illness and substance abuse. On the other hand, controlling for major mental illness, the effect of any alcohol or drug abuse was highly significant (odds ratio=26, 95 percent confidence interval=5.1 to 136, p<.001).

To address the primary goal of this study, we looked for variables among patients with a history of substance abuse that might identify a subgroup at increased risk. In particular, we hoped to find variables that might prove useful in predicting, before the onset of a major mental illness, who would later be violent. We noticed that many patients had begun abusing substances very early, in their early teens or younger. Therefore, we divided the sample into patients who had begun abusing substances before age 15—the early-onset group—and the rest of the sample. We felt that patients' recall was not precise enough to treat age of onset as a continuous variable.

As Table 3 shows, patients who had begun substance abuse before age 15 were far more likely to become violent after the onset of mental illness. We did another logistic regression analysis, controlling for major mental illness and using early onset of substance abuse in the model. We compared the ability of this model to correctly classify patients as violent or nonviolent with that of the model using adult-onset substance abuse. Both models performed well, but the area under the curve was larger for the model using early onset of substance abuse (c=.81 versus .79). The addition of other factors did not significantly improve the model's performance. Thus in this sample a premorbid characteristic—onset of substance abuse before age 15—was a better predictor of violence after the onset of mental illness than was adult-onset substance abuse.

Discussion

Consistent with previous research on violence associated with mental illness (1,3,10), substance abuse was a major risk factor in this sample of people with severe, chronic mental illness. The type of mental illness was not significant, but mental illness appeared to begin earlier for violent patients. Alternatively, because we examined only the age at first diagnosis, the latter finding might not reflect earlier onset of symptoms because violent behavior may have brought these patients to the attention of the mental health system earlier.

We were interested in whether all people with mental illness who abused substances had a similar risk of violence or whether the risk might be higher in a more homogeneous subgroup. The most interesting finding in our study was that a characteristic that preceded the development of a major mental illness by several years—the onset of alcohol or drug abuse before age 15—was the strongest risk factor for violence. This finding, if confirmed, would have important implications for how we view the relationship between substance abuse and violence among people with mental illness.

Despite the consistency of the association of substance abuse with violence, the nature of this relationship remains unclear. For people with major mental illness, both direct and indirect mechanisms have been proposed (11,17). One theory is that substance abuse causes some psychiatric patients to be violent, possibly as a result of increasing the severity of their psychotic symptoms (11). However, violence is also strongly associated with substance abuse among people without mental illness, and although alcohol or drugs may lower inhibitions, most people do not become violent when intoxicated.

Despite numerous studies, it has not been possible to clearly demonstrate that substance abuse causes violence (Reiss and Roth [18] and Miczek and associates [19] review that relationship). The best information we have about the relationship between substances and violence is for alcohol. Studies of alcoholics that include longitudinal data have found that the risk of violence is strongest when there is a history of both aggressiveness and alcohol abuse in childhood or early adolescence (19). In addition, violence has been shown to be specifically associated with the early-onset type of alcoholism (20, 21). Thus substance abuse and a tendency toward violence may both be determined by factors operating in early life.

Our finding that the risk of violence among people with mental illness is greatest when substance abuse begins before age 15 is the first evidence we are aware of that early-life antecedents are significant predictors of violence associated with adult mental illness. In a birth cohort study, Hodgins (3) found that persons with mental illness who were convicted of a crime were more likely to have abused substances in childhood or early adolescence, but no specific mention of violent crime in relation to this finding was made.

Other factors that have been reported to be associated with violence among persons with mental illness—homelessness (22), age and gender (23–25), and history of suicide attempts (26)—were not significantly more frequent in our group of violent patients if we controlled for type I error. Psychiatric diagnosis did not differentiate the violent patients from the nonviolent patients in our study, in contrast to other studies (17,24). In our retrospective study we could not assess either the severity or the type of psychotic symptoms, which have previously been found to be important risk factors (2). We also did not examine other reported risk factors, such as neurological impairment (27) and noncompliance with treatment (28). Our sample size may explain the failure to corroborate reports of other risk factors.

Overall, the contribution by people with major mental illness to the problem of violence in our society is small (1,5). However, among people receiving treatment for chronic mental illness, in which the rate of substance abuse is high (8), violence is a serious problem. Among the patients in our study, 58 percent had a history of violence since the onset of illness. If our findings are confirmed, it would be possible to identify a subgroup of persons with mental illness who abuse substances and who are at higher risk for violence.

Furthermore, our results suggest it may be possible to predict at the outset of mental illness who will be at risk for later violence based on premorbid history. This ability could have important implications for efforts to reduce the risk of violence associated with mental illness. Efforts toward the prevention and treatment of substance abuse in this patient population will be important but may not be enough. Our ability to predict, prevent, and treat violence will depend on a better understanding of the link between substance abuse and violence. An area for future study is whether the neuropsychological impairment reported to be associated with violence in the general population (29,30) and among mentally ill offenders (31,32; Fulwiler and associates, unpublished manuscript, 1997) could be related to the effects of early substance abuse on normal maturation of cognitive or neural functions.

The findings reported here cannot be generalized until they are confirmed with a larger unselected sample using structured interviews administered by investigators who are blind to the subject's history of violence. The subjects for this study were a selected group, as referrals to the community treatment team must be refractory to standard outpatient care. Also we may have misclassified some patients as nonviolent if they did not report the violent behavior and the available records were incomplete. Finally other historical information, such as age of onset and previous history of substance abuse, could also be unreliable in some cases. Finally, structured interviews were not used to make the diagnoses.

Conclusions

The rate of previous violence in the patients referred to a community treatment team serving low-income, inner-city neighborhoods in Boston was high, as was the rate of substance abuse. The most interesting finding was that a history of substance abuse beginning in late childhood or early adolescence was a better predictor than adult-onset substance abuse in discriminating violent from nonviolent patients. This finding has implications for risk assessment and management of outpatients with serious mental illness and substance abuse. Further study will be needed to determine if our finding extends to other psychiatric populations. ♦

References

1. Swanson J, Holzer C, Ganju V, et al: Violence and psychiatric disorder in the community: evidence from the Epidemiologic Catchment Area surveys. Hospital and Community Psychiatry 41:761–770, 1990
2. Link BG, Andrews HA, Cullen FT: The violent and illegal behavior of mental patients reconsidered. American Sociological Review 57:275–292, 1992
3. Hodgins S: Mental disorder, intellectual deficiency, and crime. Archives of General Psychiatry 49:476–483, 1992
4. Rabkin J: Criminal behavior of discharged mental patients: a critical review of the research. Psychological Bulletin 86:1–27, 1979
5. Monahan J: Mental disorder and violent behavior: attitudes and evidence. American Psychologist 47:511–521, 1992
6. Beck J, White K, Gage B: Emergency psychiatric assessment of violence. American Journal of Psychiatry 148:1562–1565, 1991
7. McNiel DE, Myers RS, Zeiner HK, et al: The role of violence in decisions about hospitalization from the psychiatric emergency room. American Journal of Psychiatry 149:207–212, 1992
8. Robins LN, Regier DA: Psychiatric Disorders in America. New York, Free Press, 1991
9. Lindqvist P, Allebeck P: Schizophrenia and crime: a longitudinal follow-up of 644 schizophrenics in Stockholm. British Journal of Psychiatry 157:345–350, 1990
10. Lindqvist P, Allebeck P: Schizophrenia and assaultive behavior: the role of alcohol and drug abuse. Acta Psychiatrica Scandinavia 82:191–195, 1989
11. Torrey EF: Violent behavior by individuals with serious mental illness. Hospital and Community Psychiatry 45:653–662, 1994
12. Stein L, Test M: Alternative to the hospital: a controlled study. American Journal of Psychiatry 132:517–522, 1975
13. Stein L, Test M: Alternative to mental hospital treatment: I. conceptual model, treatment program, and clinical evaluation. Archives of General Psychiatry 37:392–397, 1980
14. Diagnostic and Statistical Manual of Mental Disorders, 4th ed. Washington, DC, American Psychiatric Association, 1994
15. Shader R, Jackson A, Harmatz J, et al: Patterns of violent behavior among schizophrenic inpatients. Diseases of the Nervous System 38:13–16, 1977
16. Convit A, Isay D, Gardioma R, et al: Underreporting of physical assaults in schizophrenic inpatients. Journal of Nervous and Mental Disease 176:507–509, 1988
17. Volavka J: Neurobiology of Violence. Washington, DC, American Psychiatric Press, 1995
18. Reiss AJ Jr, Roth JA (eds): Understanding and Preventing Violence: Panel on the Understanding and Control of Violent Behavior. Washington, DC, National Academy Press, 1993
19. Miczek KA, DeBold JF, Haney M, et al: Alcohol, drugs of abuse, aggression, and violence, in Understanding and Preventing Violence, Vol 3: Social Influences. Edited by Reiss AJ Jr, Roth JA. Washington, DC, National Academy Press, 1994
20. Cloninger CR, Bohman M, Sigvardsson S: Inheritance of alcohol abuse: cross-fostering analysis of adopted men. Archives of General Psychiatry 38:861–868, 1981
21. Virkkunen M, Linnoila M: Brain serotonin, type II alcoholism, and impulsive violence. Journal of Studies on Alcohol 11(suppl):163–169, 1993
22. Martell DA, Rosner R, Harmon RB: Base-rate estimates of criminal behavior by homeless mentally ill persons in New York City. Psychiatric Services 46:596–601, 1995
23. Tardiff K, Koenigsberg H: Assaultive behavior among psychiatric outpatients. American Journal of Psychiatry 142:960–963, 1985
24. Krakowski M, Volavka J, Brizer D: Psychopathology and violence: a review of literature. Comprehensive Psychiatry 27:131–148, 1986
25. Kay S, Wolkenfeld F, Murrill L: Profiles of aggression among psychiatric patients: II. covariates and predictors. Journal of Nervous and Mental Disease 176:547–557, 1988
26. Virkkunen M, DeJong J, Bartko J, et al: Psychobiological concomitants of history of suicide attempts among violent offenders and impulsive fire setters. Archives of General Psychiatry 46:604–606, 1989
27. Krakowski M, Convit A, Jaeger J, et al: Inpatient violence: trait and state. Journal of Psychiatric Research 23:57–64, 1989
28. Bartels J, Drake R, Wallach M: Characteristic hostility in schizophrenic outpatients. Schizophrenia Bulletin 17:163–171, 1991
29. Mungas D: An empirical analysis of specific syndromes of violent behavior. Journal of Nervous and Mental Disease 171:354–361, 1983
30. Mungas D: Psychometric correlates of episodic violent behavior: a multidimensional neuropsychological approach. British Journal of Psychiatry 152:180–187, 1988
31. Krakowski M, Convit A, Jaeger J, et al: Neurological impairment in violent schizophrenic inpatients. American Journal of Psychiatry 146:849–853, 1989
32. Krakowski MI, Czobor P: Clinical symptoms, neurological impairment, and prediction of violence in psychiatric inpatients. Hospital and Community Psychiatry 45:700–705, 1994

Command Hallucinations and the Prediction of Dangerousness

John Junginger, Ph.D.

Objectives: Recent studies have supported the belief that command hallucinations can induce dangerous behavior. This study tried to replicate previous findings that compliance with the command was associated with delusions related to hallucinations and the ability to identify the hallucinated voice. This study also assessed the association between compliance and the dangerousness of the command, chronicity of illness, a diagnosis of schizophrenia, and past compliance with hallucinated commands. *Methods:* The most recent command hallucination reported by 93 psychiatric inpatients was rated for level of dangerousness and level of compliance with the command. *Results:* Subjects who experienced less dangerous commands or who could identify the hallucinated voice reported higher levels of compliance, although reported compliance with more dangerous commands was not uncommon. Commands experienced in the hospital were less dangerous than those experienced elsewhere and tended to be specific to the hospital environment. Subjects were less likely to comply with commands experienced in the hospital. *Conclusions:* Based on their self-reports, psychiatric patients who experience command hallucinations are at risk for dangerous behavior. Ability to identify the hallucinated voice is a fairly reliable predictor of reported compliance. Level of dangerousness resulting from compliance with command hallucinations may be a function of the patient's environment.

There seems to be a developing opinion among researchers, although by no means a consensus (1,2), that command hallucinations can induce dangerous or criminal behavior among psychiatric patients. Psychiatric textbooks have expressed this opinion for some time (3,4), but empirical support has been presented only recently.

For example, Rogers and associates (5) found that 20 of 25 forensic inpatients (80 percent) who recently experienced a command hallucination reported that they had complied with a command in the recent past. Even more notable was that 14 patients (56 percent) reported that they had complied with a command hallucination "with unquestioning obedience" at least once, and 11 patients (44 percent) reported that they complied "on a frequent or very frequent basis."

Although Rogers and associates found that the majority of hallucinated commands had some criminal content, the respective rates of compliance with criminal and noncriminal commands were not assessed. Nevertheless, they concluded that command hallucinations exert considerable control over the actions of chronic forensic psychiatric patients and may have a substantial influence on criminal behavior.

In an earlier study, I assessed the most recent command hallucination of 51 psychiatric inpatients and outpatients and found that 20 patients (39 percent) reported that they had complied with that command (6).

More relevant to the issue of the risk posed by command hallucinations was the finding that eight patients (16 percent) reported compliance with a dangerous command. In addition, patients who could identify the hallucinated voice as a fairly specific person or entity and patients who had delusions related to hallucinations were significantly more likely to report compliance. Dangerousness of the command did not appear to be a factor in compliance. However, seven patients (14 percent) who reported harmless commands claimed that they could not recall whether they had complied; thus compliance with harmless commands may have been underreported.

Given an association between command hallucinations and patients' reports of dangerous or criminal behavior, further investigation is needed to identify which patients are at risk for

---

When this paper was published Dr. Junginger was visiting professor in the department of psychology at the State University of New York at Binghamton. From the September 1995 issue of Psychiatric Services *(volume 46, pages 911–914).*

compliance. Earlier findings suggest that the patient's being able to identify the hallucinated voice and the presence of a delusion related to hallucinations increase the likelihood of compliance (6). In addition, several other variables seem to be consistent with clinical notions about patients who comply with command hallucinations.

For example, McNiel (1) claimed that the risk for assaultive behavior is "obviously higher" for a patient with a history of behaving violently in response to hallucinations. Benjamin (7) described several relationships between patients and their hallucinated voices that could indicate that compliance is a function of chronicity and, by implication, a diagnosis of schizophrenia. Finally, in light of possible underreporting of compliance with harmless commands in a previous study (6), the dangerousness of the command continues to be of interest as a variable that may influence compliance.

The study reported here tried to replicate previous findings that compliance with hallucinated commands is associated with the patient's having delusions related to hallucinations and being able to identify the hallucinated voice. Associations between compliance and dangerousness of the command, a diagnosis of schizophrenia, chronicity of the patient's illness, and past compliance with hallucinated commands were also assessed.

Methods
Subjects
Ninety-three subjects were selected from among approximately 370 inpatients at three hospitals providing short-term psychiatric treatment. These subjects reported in a preliminary screening interview that they had a history of at least one command hallucination.

Twenty of the 93 subjects (21.5 percent) reported experiencing a command hallucination the day of their assessment, 71 subjects (76.3 percent) within the previous two weeks, 85 subjects (91.4 percent) within the previous year, and 93 subjects (100 percent) within the previous two years. The majority of subjects (61.3 percent) were assigned a diagnosis of schizophrenia based on their responses to the Structured Clinical Interview for DSM-III-R (SCID) (8).

Fifty-one subjects (54.8 percent) were male. Fifty-four subjects (58.1 percent) were black, and 39 were white (41.9 percent). The mean±SD number of years of education for the entire sample was 10.4±8.9. They had a mean of 6.9±6.2 psychiatric hospitalizations, although data on hospitalization were considered marginally reliable due to numerous discrepancies between subjects' reports and hospital records.

Procedure
During a semistructured interview, subjects were asked to describe verbatim what the hallucinated voice said during their most recent command hallucination. Subjects were asked whether and how they complied with that command and to identify the hallucinated voice. They also were asked whether and how they had complied with hallucinated commands in the past.

Subjects were assessed for the presence of delusions during their most recent command hallucination by asking them specific questions about delusions taken from the SCID

Command hallucinations experienced in the hospital tended to be specific to the hospital environment or could be complied with in the hospital as easily as outside it. No subjects reported experiencing commands to shoot someone with a gun while in the hospital.

(8). Subjects who reported delusions at the time of their most recent command hallucination were asked to describe the delusions in detail and provide evidence for the beliefs. Delusions were considered to be related to hallucinations if patients referred to verbal hallucinations as evidence for their delusions (6).

After the semistructured interview, 88 subjects (94.6 percent) answered general questions about their social and sexual history that were drawn from an instrument for measuring premorbid adjustment of patients with schizophrenia (9). The instrument is used to rate patients' social and sexual functioning before onset of the disorder on a scale from 0, better functioning, to 6, poorer functioning. Higher scores have been shown to identify patients with schizophrenia who had poorer prognoses (9). For the analysis reported here, these ratings were used as a general estimate of the chronicity of subjects' illnesses.

A research assistant who was blind to the study's purpose and to subjects' impressions of the identities of the hallucinated voices read subjects' descriptions of their most recent command hallucination, whether and how they complied with that command, and whether and how they had complied with such commands in the past. She then rated the dangerousness of the most recent command, the level of compliance with that command, and the level of compliance with past commands. The ratings of dangerousness were made on a 3-point scale on which 0 indicated not at all dangerous; 1, somewhat dangerous; and 2, very dangerous. Compliance with commands was rated on a 3-point scale on which 0 indicated no compliance; 1, partial compliance; and 2, full compliance.

The reliability of the research assistant's ratings was assessed by calculating intraclass correlational coefficients (10) between her ratings and ratings done independently by me. Separate coefficients were calculated for the ratings of dangerousness of the most recent command hallucination, compliance with the most recent command hallucination, and compliance with past commands. Coefficients of .95 or greater were found for all three measures, indicating excellent reliability for single raters using these methods.

Results

The mean rating of compliance with the most recent command hallucination was .99±.94 (95 percent confidence interval=.80 to 1.18); the mean rating of dangerousness of the most recent command hallucination was 1.14±.93 (95 percent CI=.95 to 1.33). These findings indicated that subjects as a group could be described as reporting partial compliance with somewhat dangerous commands.

Twenty-five subjects experienced their most recent command hallucination while hospitalized. The mean± SD rating of compliance with commands in the hospital was .88±.93. For the 68 subjects who reported experiencing their most recent command outside the hospital, the mean rating for compliance was 1.03±.91. The difference in these mean ratings of compliance was not statistically significant.

The mean±SD rating of dangerousness was .72±.94 for commands experienced in the hospital and 1.29±.90 for commands experienced outside the hospital. The difference in these means was significant (t= 2.74, df=91, p<.01), indicating that subjects who were in the hospital at the time of their most recent command hallucination reported less dangerous commands. Relevant to this finding was the observation that commands experienced in the hospital tended to be specific to the hospital environment or could be complied with in the hospital as easily as outside it. For example, no subjects reported experiencing commands to shoot someone with a gun in the hospital. Thus subjects' psychotic experiences seemed to have adapted to the more restrictive hospital environment.

Despite the marginal reliability of the data on previous hospitalizations, the measure of premorbid functioning was significantly correlated with the number of psychiatric hospitalizations (r=.23, p<.05) but with no other subject characteristics that we measured. This finding supported the use of the measure of premorbid functioning as an estimate of chronicity of illness.

Table 1

Level of patients' reported compliance with hallucinated commands, by level of dangerousness of the command and whether the patient identified the hallucinated voice

Level of compliance	Level of dangerousness[1]				Identified voice[2]	
	Not at all (N=34)	Somewhat (N=12)	Very (N=47)	All levels (N=93)	Yes (N=64)	No (N=29)
None	9	3	29	41	22	19
Partial	1	4	7	12	8	4
Full	24	5	11	40	34	6

[1] $\chi^2=23.55$, df=4, p<.001
[2] $\chi^2=9.30$, df=2, p<.01

The score on the measure of premorbid functioning and five other variables were entered as predictors of compliance in a multiple regression analysis. The five other variables were presence of a delusion related to hallucinations, whether the hallucinated voice was identified, diagnosis of schizophrenia, and ratings of the dangerousness of the most recent command hallucination and of the highest level of past compliance. The rating of compliance with the most recent command hallucination was entered as the outcome variable. The analysis involved data from 88 subjects (94.6 percent) for whom all measures were completed. The predictor variables were entered into the regression equation in a stepwise, forward manner. The p value for variables to enter the equation and to be removed from the equation was .05.

Dangerousness of the command (F=13.62, df=1,86, p<.001) and an identified hallucinated voice (F=6.14, df=1,86, p<.02) entered a multiple regression model that significantly predicted compliance (F=10.27, df= 2,85, p<.001). This result indicated that subjects who reported relatively less dangerous commands and subjects who could identify the hallucinated voice reported higher levels of compliance with their most recent command hallucination.

The results of t tests reported earlier indicated that subjects who experienced their most recent command hallucination while hospitalized reported less dangerous commands, but not higher levels of compliance, than subjects who experienced their most recent command hallucination outside the hospital. In light of the prominent effect of dangerousness in the multiple regression analysis, analysis of covariance was used to statistically control the effect of dangerousness on compliance for commands inside and outside the hospital. The results of this analysis showed that subjects who were in the hospital at the time of their most recent command hallucination reported lower levels of compliance (F=4.16, df= 1,90, p<.05), another indication of the modifying effect of the hospital environment.

Table 1 shows the numbers of subjects who reported each of the three levels of compliance with their most recent command hallucination, grouped by three levels of dangerousness of the command and by whether the subject identified the hallucinated voice. The effects of the dangerousness of the command and identifying the hallucinated voice can be clearly seen. Of the 34 subjects whose command hallucinations were judged to be not at all dangerous, 25 subjects (73.5 percent) reported at least partial compliance with the command, compared with 27 of the 59 subjects (45.8 percent) whose command hallucinations were judged to be somewhat or very dangerous. Similarly, 42 of 64 subjects (65.6 percent) who identified the hallucinated voice reported at least partial compliance with the command, compared with only ten of 29 subjects (34.5 percent) who could not identify the hallucinated voice.

Potentially more informative for the prediction of dangerous behavior was whether the subject identified the hallucinated voice and the level of reported compliance across the three levels of dangerousness. In these subgroups, the effect of dangerousness was again evident. Among subjects who identified their hallucinated voice, 22 of the 26 subjects (84.6 percent) whose commands were judged not at all dangerous reported at least partial compliance, compared with 20 of 37 subjects (54.1 percent) whose commands were judged somewhat or very dangerous. Note, however, that these respective percentages of compliance are well above those reported for commands characterized by dangerousness alone (73.5 percent for commands that were not at all dangerous and 45.8 percent for commands that were somewhat or very dangerous) due to the effect of whether the hallucinated voice identified.

The effect of identifying the hallucinated voice also was evident in the most dangerous behavior reported in the sample. Of subjects whose commands were judged to be very dangerous, nine of 28 subjects (32.1 percent) who identified the hallucinated voice reported full compliance, compared with only two of 19 subjects (10.5 percent) who could not identify the hallucinated voice. In all but two cases, reports of full compliance with very dangerous commands were independently verified by hospital records.

Discussion

Like previous research (5,6), this study found that reported compliance with command hallucinations is not uncommon: 52 of 93 subjects (55.9 percent) reported at least partial compliance with their most recent command hallucination, and 40 of 93 (43 percent) reported full compliance. This latter percentage of full compliance is similar to that found in an earlier study using a dichotomous measure of compliance (6).

It should be recognized, however, that the issue of compliance with command hallucinations cannot be meaningfully addressed without considering the type of behavior specified by the command. This study showed significant differences between subjects' level of compliance with dangerous commands and their compliance with harmless commands, compliance being much more likely for commands judged relatively less dangerous. This finding clearly indicates that researchers should continue to make the distinction between harmless and dangerous commands when assessing and reporting compliance rates.

This study replicated a previous finding of an association between whether the subject identified the hallucinated voice and the reported level of compliance (6). What now seems fairly reliable is that a patient who gives an identity to a hallucinated voice should be considered at somewhat greater risk for compliance than a patient who cannot identify the hallucinated voice.

Of course, the ultimate danger of compliance is a function of the dangerousness of the command. In this study, the apparent adaptation of the subjects' psychotic experience to the more restrictive hospital environment raises the possibility that environments outside the hospital could be modified to discourage development of dangerous command hallucinations. Such modifications could involve, for example, limiting the patient's exposure to weapons. For a psychotic patient, the danger posed by weapons is that they could become integrated into the patient's psychotic experience.

Conclusions

If the reports of psychiatric patients are taken at face value, they are at risk for dangerous behavior if the hallucinated voice commands such behavior. Patients who give an identity to the hallucinated voice are at somewhat greater risk for compliance with the hallucinated command.

An additional consideration when assessing risk of dangerous behavior is the patient's environment. This study's findings suggest that dangerousness is a function not only of various characteristics of a patient and his or her illness, but also of the particular characteristics of the patient's psychotic experience that are based in the patient's environment. What should concern us, of course, is that hospital-based assessment of risk may be unreliable. Rather, it may be the posthospital environment that determines the dangerousness of command hallucinations and thus the patient's potential for violent and criminal behavior. ♦

Acknowledgments

This study was supported by grant MH–47005 from the National Institute of Mental Health. The author thanks Shannon Holcomb, Sheryl Williams, M.S.W., Judith Levy, M.A., Roy Allen, Ph.D., Jay Pennington, M.D., Elisa Phelan, M.A., Betti Giles, M.S.W., Martha Corley, and Heather Kilpatrick for their help with data collection and analysis.

References

1. McNiel D: Hallucinations and violence, in Violence and Mental Disorder: Developments in Risk Assessment. Edited by Monahan J, Steadman H. Chicago, University of Chicago Press, 1994
2. Hellerstein D, Frosch W, Koenigsberg HW: The clinical significance of command hallucinations. American Journal of Psychiatry 144:219–221, 1987
3. Lehman H: Clinical features of schizophrenia, in Comprehensive Textbook of Psychiatry, 1st ed. Edited by Freedman A, Kaplan H. Baltimore, Williams & Wilkins, 1967
4. Kolb L: Modern Clinical Psychiatry, 9th ed. Philadelphia, Saunders, 1977
5. Rogers R, Gillis J, Turner R, et al: The clinical presentation of command hallucinations in a forensic population. American Journal of Psychiatry 147:1304–1307, 1990
6. Junginger J: Predicting compliance with command hallucinations. American Journal of Psychiatry 147:245–247, 1990
7. Benjamin L: Is chronicity a function of the relationship between the person and the auditory hallucination? Schizophrenia Bulletin 15:291–309, 1989
8. Spitzer R, Williams J, Gibbon M, et al: Structured Clinical Interview for DSM-III-R, Patient Edition. Washington, DC, American Psychiatric Press, 1990
9. Harris J: An abbreviated form of the Phillips Rating Scale of Premorbid Adjustment in Schizophrenia. Journal of Abnormal Psychology 84:129–137, 1975
10. Shrout P, Fleiss J: Intraclass correlations: uses in assessing rater reliability. Psychological Bulletin 86:420–428, 1979